DR. DENESE'S
SECRETS FOR
AGELESS SKIN

DR. DENESE'S
SECRETS FOR AGELESS SKIN

Younger Skin in 8 Weeks

ADRIENNE DENESE, M.D., Ph.D.

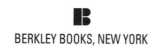
BERKLEY BOOKS, NEW YORK

THE BERKLEY PUBLISHING GROUP
Published by the Penguin Group
Penguin Group (USA) Inc.
375 Hudson Street, New York, New York 10014, USA
Penguin Group (Canada), 10 Alcorn Avenue, Toronto, Ontario M4V 3B2, Canada
(a division of Pearson Penguin Canada Inc.)
Penguin Books Ltd., 80 Strand, London WC2R 0RL, England
Penguin Group Ireland, 25 St. Stephen's Green, Dublin 2, Ireland (a division of Penguin Books Ltd.)
Penguin Group (Australia), 250 Camberwell Road, Camberwell, Victoria 3124, Australia
(a division of Pearson Australia Group Pty. Ltd.)
Penguin Books India Pvt. Ltd., 11 Community Centre, Panchsheel Park, New Delhi—110 017, India
Penguin Group (NZ), Cnr. Airborne and Rosedale Roads, Albany, Auckland 1310, New Zealand
(a division of Pearson New Zealand Ltd.)
Penguin Books (South Africa) (Pty.) Ltd., 24 Sturdee Avenue, Rosebank, Johannesburg 2196, South Africa

Penguin Books Ltd., Registered Offices: 80 Strand, London WC2R 0RL, England

DR. DENESE'S SECRETS FOR AGELESS SKIN

This book is an original publication of The Berkley Publishing Group.

Copyright © 2005 by Denese Products, LLC.

Botox® is a registered trademark of Allergan.
StriVectin SD® is a registered trademark of Klein-Becker.

First edition: March 2005

Library of Congress Cataloging-in-Publication Data

Denese, Adrienne.
    Dr. Denese's secrets for ageless skin : younger skin in 8 weeks / Adrienne Denese.
        p.   cm.
    ISBN: 0-425-20410-3
        1. Skin—Care and hygiene.   I. Title

    RL87.D46   2005
    646.7'26—dc22   2004066025

PRINTED IN THE UNITED STATES OF AMERICA

10   9   8   7   6   5   4   3   2   1

PUBLISHER'S NOTE: Every effort has been made to ensure that the information contained in this book is complete and accurate. However, neither the publisher nor the author is engaged in rendering professional advice or services to the individual reader. The ideas, procedures, and suggestions contained in this book are not intended as a substitute for consulting with your physician. All matters regarding your health require medical supervision. Neither the author nor the publisher shall be liable or responsible for any loss or damage allegedly arising from any information or suggestion in this book.

Dedicated to the memory of my Father and Grandmother,
the two most important people in my life.

ACKNOWLEDGMENTS

My thanks to Lee Quarfoot for her assistance with the manuscript. I want to give special thanks to my editor, Jane Stine, and to my friends Ken and Linda Raasch for their invaluable help and guidance in converting the idea of this book into a reality.

CONTENTS

FOREWORD

"Dr. Denese, what's your secret? How do you stay so young? How do you keep your skin so ageless?"

I have been asked those questions many times. My answer is always the same. *My secret is science.*

I have always believed that scientific knowledge can conquer nearly any skin problem. Scientific knowledge is the keystone of my success in helping my patients achieve results in fighting the effects of aging. Medical science, not marketing, has guided me as I created my skin-care products. But even before that, it was scientific knowledge that helped me escape the bleakness of my childhood in communist Hungary.

I was born in Hungary during the height of communism. Life was bleak for a kid during that time—no TV, no fashion, no shopping, no parties, no dances, no movies, no games . . . nothing.

We had two hours of television broadcasting a night, one channel only, and it was mostly heavily censored news. We had one hour of pop music a week, on Saturdays between three and four o'clock. Life as we knew it stopped for that hour—we were glued to the radio listening to the Beatles, in awe for that one magical hour each Saturday afternoon.

Shopping was not much fun either. The stores carried a choice of one kind of skirt: pleated in navy. Your choice was to buy one or not to buy one. Blouses were white or yellow and they rarely had the right size for a teenager, so shopping was out.

Food shopping was equally unexciting. You cannot even fathom what a grocery shop looked like during the height of communism. I lived next door to one as a child and I went there at least twice a day, so I remember it as if it was yesterday. It was a simple rectangular store with no middle aisles since there was nothing to display. No fruits and no vegetables except potatoes, cabbage, and onions. One wall was covered with uniform bags of government-brand flour and sugar. The opposite wall had bags of salt, a few bottles of oil and vinegar. There was one brand of soap and a single brand of shampoo and one brand of toothpaste and Vaseline—no creams, no makeup, no deodorant, no laundry detergent, nothing else. In the front of the store, chunks of lard and one type of cheese lined the small shelf. The milk and butter came at eight in the morning. I knew that because a line immediately formed outside the store and stretched around the corner until all the goods were sold. Bread came at noon. The line was even longer then. When I was five, it was my job to run and stand in line as soon as possible because bread sold out as fast as it came. It may sound odd, but I loved standing in line for bread. At five years old, it made me feel like a real contributor to the household.

My grandmother was perhaps the most influential person in my life. She was solid, predictable, never left the house, worked incessantly, and was always there for me. She got up at five every day, chopped wood, fed all the wood- and coal-burning stoves in the house (there was no central heating), fed the chickens and pigs, collected the eggs, cleaned the house, made pasta from flour and water, cooked, baked, made elaborate meals, did laundry by hand (no washing machine), and tended to a large vegetable garden and about fifty apple trees. At night, she peeled piles of apples for jam and pie, or knitted sweaters for me. I remember watching her hands, amazed at how they never seemed to stop.

Whatever was soft, nurturing, and pleasant in my life came from my grandmother. She also taught me the value of hard work. She used to say that there is never enough time in the day—and absolutely no time to be idle! She made sure I was always busy and always learning.

My father grew up before communism took hold in Budapest, a privileged child of a prominent tax lawyer. He was sixteen when the Second World War broke out. He lived through the bombing of Budapest and the bombing of Dresden in Germany. He walked home from Germany through Austria to Hungary. He literally came home on foot at the end of the war, by himself. He was only nineteen years old. He never talked about what he saw, but he never quite recovered from the experience. He became a bitter, angry, opinionated man and suffered from depression for most of his life. His emotional burden must have been nearly unbearable. However, he was a very intelligent man. He read everything he could get his hands on, and whatever he read, he remembered. He was remarkably worldly, well informed, and razor sharp in his political predictions. He taught me the value of education and always encouraged me to study, which I did.

My mother had the face of an angel, and she acted like one. She was a national sports champion in short-distance sprinting and high jumping. She trained incessantly—that is all she knew how to do. She was not very good in school, and was never very knowledgeable or well informed about world affairs. But she was charming, charitable, naive, kind, and selfless.

Whenever I think of my mother, one particular incident always comes to mind. We had a tall, wrought-iron gate in front of our house in the small town where I was born. It was a well-made iron piece, ornate with many flowers and about two stories high. It dated back well before communism. I was about five years old when I finally figured out how to climb to the very top. When I tried to show my grandmother how well I could climb, she nearly fainted and ordered me never to do it again. My aunt, a frail, refined, white-haired lady, had an even more violent reaction. When I showed my mother, I expected something very similar. However, she remained calm, applauded when I got to the top of the gate, and told me, "As long as you hold on to something with one hand, as long as you hold on really tight, you can climb up as high as you want."

This advice guided me through some tough times. Even today when I face new challenges, when I feel insecure, her words come back to me. She taught me to be careful but not to be afraid to take a risk.

So I climbed up all the gates and all the fences, barn roofs, and toolsheds I could find. Holding on really tight at all times with at least one hand, I felt as if I could master nearly anything. I proudly stood in line for milk and butter in the mornings. I brought home the bread at noon every day. I felt that I was making a great difference in the house, and I had not even started grade school yet. It helps to live in a small world, where you feel you can master it all, at least for a few happy years.

When I was nine years old, my aunt began to make her famous bee pollen face cream for the ladies in the neighborhood. It was a family recipe and promised smoother, firmer skin. Of course I was right there "helping" her. She measured and mixed the ingredients, and I stirred the pots as they heated on the stove.

During the height of communism, any kind of private enterprise was strictly forbidden, so we had to work behind closed doors and drawn curtains. Given the selection in the grocery store, you can imagine the enthusiastic reception this cream received. Soon my aunt's cream became so well known that hundreds of women came to buy it. They came at night, in secrecy, knocking on the kitchen window.

Eventually the authorities took notice. The secret police came one night, confiscated all the cream, and shut us down. My aunt just narrowly escaped going to jail. I will never forget that night. It was frightening when the police came, but when I look back it's the fun of helping my aunt make the cream—and seeing the enthusiasm of the local ladies as they calmored to buy it—that comes to mind. That's what has stayed with me all these years.

Except for the bright, brief, and exciting episode of cream-making, most of my childhood memories are of studying. Life was bleak during communism.

There were no dances and no parties because there was rarely music to dance to. Western records were a rarity and we did not have decent sound systems. Plus the police were not keen on the idea of Western pop music blasting into the night. The movies were mostly about Hungarian peasants and industrial workers, showing how happy and hopeful their lives had become now that communism had arrived. Believe me, I really was better off studying.

I studied physics, chemistry, biology, Latin, English, and German with great enthusiasm. I took great comfort in the fact that at least these textbooks were not rewritten by the ruling party, unlike our history or literature texts. Studying made me feel that I had a connection to the world beyond communism. It was a world I knew little about, but I knew it existed—or at least I hoped it did.

I completed a Ph.D. in neuroscience at the very early age of twenty-two and made plans to come to America and study medicine. My father spent his entire life's savings on a one-way airplane ticket to New York. He had $40 left, so he gave it to me for spending money.

I came to the United States by myself at age twenty-three, not knowing a single soul here. No relatives, no friends, no acquaintances, nothing. It was the single most difficult thing I had ever done, but I felt there was no choice. I could not see myself listening to news or reading books and newspapers rewritten by the ruling party for the rest of my life.

It still gives me chills to remember saying good-bye to my family at the small town train station. I remember my grandmother struggling with tears, I'd never seen her cry before. We all thought we were seeing each other for the last time.

When I arrived in New York, I stayed with a pen pal and supported myself with menial jobs. Then, after about eight months of unimaginable struggle for survival, I received a postdoctoral fellowship at the University of Pennsylvania. It did not pay anything at first, but it gave me room and board and access to a medical library that was beyond compare. The library was open until midnight every day, even on Sundays. I was fascinated by this because in Hungary the university library closed at 6:00 P.M. without exception. I spent endless hours at the Penn library, trying to make up for lost time.

The head of the department at Penn was baffled by me at first. He had never seen anyone who asked for nothing and worked around the clock. I guess he had never been to Hungary. He liked me a lot, and eventually we published many scientific papers together, detailing how the right and the left sides of the brain differ from each other and how the brain organizes sustained attention (vigilance) response.

One day, I was invited to give a lecture at the Neurology Department at Harvard Medical School on the brain studies we conducted at Penn. When I got the letter of invitation, I could not believe it and I was sure that the letter was addressed to the wrong person. I called, learned that it was meant for me, and terror set in. I studied day and night, wrote the lecture, memorized it, including the jokes, and on a Tuesday, very early in the morning, went to Boston. I was in a bad state; I was so nervous I vomited in the taxicab on the way to Harvard. When I arrived, I went to the bathroom, cleaned up, looked in the mirror, and something clicked in my head. I realized I couldn't be in worse shape, so I really had nothing to lose.

The lecture went very well. Fifty people, all in white coats, clapped enthusiastically. The head of the department, a man of few words, stood and called the ideas extremely interesting and offered me a fellowship at Harvard then and there. I accepted, mostly because I was hopelessly in love with him by the end of the evening.

The love story went nowhere, but Harvard was great. It taught me how little I really knew and spurred me to go to medical school.

When the time came, I applied to one medical school only, Cornell, in Manhattan. For those who know anything about applying to medical school, this move is nearly suicidal. Normally, you apply to about twenty and hope to get into one or two. I had no idea that this is the way it is done. Luckily, I got into Cornell. I received a full scholarship to study medicine.

I was the oldest in my class (age thirty-two) and felt totally out of place among my bright, young Ivy League classmates. Many of them were a decade younger, born in the United States, bred on sports, TV, pop music, and fast food. I was a good student, but it did not come as easily to me as it did to my younger classmates. For the first time, I began to experience the uneasy feeling that comes with getting older. So in an effort to retain my youth for as long as possible, I developed an overwhelming interest in research intended to control the aging process.

After completing medical school and residency at Cornell Medical College at New York Hospital Medical Center, I opened an anti-aging medical practice in Manhattan, a few blocks from my alma mater.

All the wise ones told me: nobody opens a practice right after residency; you are sure to go out of business with the rent you have to pay. Quite possible, I thought, but if I can just make enough to pay rent . . . even if nothing more . . . I would find it so fascinating to see people and advise them on how to cope with what we think of as the inevitable: aging. So, with some trepidation, I opened anyway. It must have been an idea whose time had come, because a few months later the *New York Times* wrote a two-page article about my clinic. Two days later, I was on *Good Morning America* and a few weeks after that on *20/20,* in a segment exclusively dedicated to the subject of anti-aging. My success confirmed what I have always believed: Growing old gracefully is no longer an option in our world.

Today we live longer than ever and, from a historical perspective, enter the prime of our lives much later than ever. We start out with a prolonged childhood and continue with a prolonged education. Then there's an intense career-building phase, a prolonged mate selection phase, followed by delayed child rearing. When middle age sets in, we often find ourselves in the most demanding, stressful, active, and productive stage of our lives, only to realize that we *now* are lacking the mental energy, focus, and physical stamina of youth.

We are trying to live a younger person's life in a middle-age body, which leads to a critical question: How can we postpone the start of middle age?

This is no longer a question of vanity. It is a question of survival.

In my practice at the Manhattan Anti-Aging Clinic in New York City, I have seen hundreds, if not thousands, of women and men seeking to ward off aging. Interestingly enough, at the end of the conversation they all settle on the issue of skin. "What can we do for my skin?" they ask.

I've seen all the ways that skin is assaulted—by time, sun, and living in a hectic world full of environmental toxins and stress. I've heard the stories of men and women who have been shocked at their own reflections in the mirror. For many of us, the awareness of our passage from young adulthood to middle age often comes as a sudden surprise. "How did that happen overnight?" we might wonder about the crow's-feet around our eyes, deepening furrows down our cheeks, or a feathering of lines along the lips.

I've witnessed these reactions to the visible signs of aging. And I've seen men and women who have achieved remarkable improvement in the appearance of their skin. Through my work, I've observed the proof that we do not have to age like the generations before us, and plastic surgery is not the only way to hold back the aging process.

It's taken me many years of medical practice to crystallize what really works for the skin. I am not only a medical doctor who specializes in anti-aging, I am also one of the very few women doctors and one of the only female scientists in the field. I bring to skin-care science my own experience and the experiences of the women I treat. I have counseled a great many women on how to fight the effects of aging. Each of my patients has told me their stories, and I know what women need to look their best. By drawing on the medical breakthroughs of the past few decades and on the development of new treatments and potent new ingredients, along with my experiences helping my patients to reverse the signs of aging, I've created a powerful program to repair and rejuvenate your skin in eight weeks. I've also developed an ongoing regimen to keep the radiance of timeless beauty into your forties, fifties, sixties, and beyond.

With proper care, skin that continues to look, feel, and act young and healthy can be yours, no matter how many candles there are on your birthday cake.

In today's world of skin-care products and treatment opinions, you need more than just a treatment program and a list of active ingredients; you also need knowledge to recognize false promises and to navigate the world of beauty, where hundreds, even thousands, of dollars can be spent without any delivery of desired results.

What I call the "skin-care conspiracy" is under way in department stores, spas, and at cosmetics counters across America. In this book I'll reveal my secrets for ageless skin. By combining new knowledge about the revolution in anti-aging treatments with my program, and with a lifestyle of healthy living, you can have a fabulous complexion for the rest of your life.

CHAPTER ONE

THE SKIN-CARE CONSPIRACY

The science of anti-aging has seen radical changes in the last decade. New discoveries have led to advances that make younger-looking skin attainable. Yet American women spend $4.3 billion a year on skin-care products that simply do *not* work.

Why? Because for decades, time has stood still at the cosmetics counter. Despite the many products promising the latest ingredients, many of us are still treating our skin exactly as our mothers did twenty, thirty, or forty years ago. And we are getting pretty much the same disappointing results. The latest and greatest ingredients and claims so prominently displayed on the latest and "greatest" expensive cream jars are often nothing more than cleverly worded promises that do not deliver yet again. The nutritional and vitamin supplement industry has made great strides formulating superior products, educating consumers, and creating industry standards that force companies to deliver the highest-quality products to the market. Unfortunately, the skin-care industry has yet to follow suit.

Let me ask you a question: Are you younger than your mother was at your age?

The answer is invariably yes.

Why would this be? Are your nutritional practices, your vitamin intake, your exercise habits, your sun exposure, and your smoking/drinking awareness different from your mother's?

Yes, again. Today's women are far more aware of what is right for the body than the previous generation, who bought their vitamins at the supermarket, were satisfied with meeting the minimum RDA vitamin requirements, and who smoked, did little exercise, got a tan as soon as summer began, spent three weeks baking at the beach each summer, and used tanning lamps for the winter.

Our level of sophistication about nutrition and fitness has changed dramatically over the past twenty-five years. The nutrition and fitness industries have kept pace with this new sophistication: There are gyms at every corner and vitamin shops selling megadoses of vitamins that would have been unimaginable to our parents and grandparents. Remember how the standard dosage for vitamin C used to be 50 mg per day? Today most people take ten or twenty times that amount.

The vitamin/nutrition industry became resigned to the idea that the right amount of a vitamin will do more for the body than some minimal amount that had been previously designated as the necessary daily requirement. Granted, it cost more to provide more, but people liked getting more and came to expect it. Slowly, the new attitude became the standard in the vitamin industry, and the anti-aging revolution began to take place.

These same changes are not taking place as quickly in the cosmetics industry. The truth is that the skin needs the same nutrients, antioxidants, and megadoses of vitamins as the rest of the body. Yet your skin is shortchanged with a mixture of oil and water and a lovely smell in a stunning jar presented to you by a beautiful twenty-year-old face.

The vitamins and nutrients your skin needs, the ingredients that are prominently displayed on the packaging and advertisements, are often present in minuscule quantities in the jar. Why aren't adequate quantities added to the products? Well, many of these ingredients are quite expensive. Others may feel irritating to the skin and the companies may be concerned about high returns. Either way, including enough key ingredients will cost the companies money—in higher manufacturing costs or from returns, which can affect their profit margin.

The skin-care industry works at an extremely high profit margin, far higher than the food, the car, or the clothing industries. Based on these high margins, the cosmetics companies are almost always profitable. Most of the company's expenditure goes for promotion and advertising. If enough money is spent on advertising, the product will be sold in adequate numbers. It may be sold only once to a specific customer; nevertheless, it will be sold in high volume, which yields high profits. The companies are making money, so why should they change?

Let me say it now: The idea of one miracle cream that feels good and is able to deliver profound changes to the appearance of your skin is nothing but a scientific fallacy. For one thing, there is no one product—no matter how expensive—that can do it all. It takes several steps of daily skin care to deliver results. Further, some of the steps will not feel good. It may tingle, it may cause irritation temporarily and it is not pleasant in the traditional skin-care sense.

It is my impression that the public is beginning to understand this idea and is becoming more and more open to a change. It is the skin-care industry that is slow to change.

I have had the opportunity to hear the conversations of many high-level executives in the cosmetics industry. They see their job as threefold:

- to keep the cost of the expensive and effective key ingredients and the cost of production in general under strict control

- to word the skin-care claims on the bottle carefully, to stay within legal boundaries

- to promote the new release in many magazines, not just in the form of ads but also in actual, objective-sounding editorial articles about the merits of the new release

When skin-care executives decide it is time for a new cream, they go to a manufacturer and say something like, "I have a budget of eighty cents per jar for a cream. What new ingredient do you have with an interesting story that fits this budget?" It is common knowledge in the industry that this is exactly how most new projects get their start. Their concerns are about marketing and, above all, staying within the almighty budget.

In my opinion, the cosmetics industry has the order wrong. When I create a new product for my skin-care line project, my first concern is using the newest, most effective, scientifically tested ingredients that actually make a significant difference in the skin. Then I ask, "What is the maximum that we can put into the product to make it really effective?" I never ask about the cost first because I don't want to be unduly influenced by it. I can't worry about the cost because we *cannot* cut corners on the active ingredient. If the active ingredient is compromised, so is the product. To me, the active ingredient is the *untouchable.* Anything else can bend—the promotion or the packaging—but *not what is inside the jar.* If we have to spend less on promotion, I am not concerned, because if the product is good, my happy and excited customers will do the selling for me. This approach has been working well for me so far, but I am definitely in the minority in the industry.

The "skin-care conspiracy" is the hidden truth inside the multibillion-dollar skin-care industry: Precious few of the claims that are made about the products out there are true. All claims are within legal boundaries because they are based on effective ingredients that are in the bottle. But the question is, at what percentage are these ingredients present in the bottle? At a percentage that fits a remarkably frugal budget, or at a percentage that can actually deliver results? There is a huge difference between these two percentages, and most cosmetics companies pay no mind to this fact.

THE PERCENTAGE GAME: "FEEL GOOD" VS. "LOOK GOOD" SKIN CARE

Back in the 1950s and '60s, the days of "cold creams," the most that skin-care manufacturers could provide were glorified moisturizers, pitched to consumers on the appeal of beautiful models, glamorous photography, and value of a brand. Today there are truly effective ingredients (beginning with retinol, synthetic forms of vitamin A that were developed in the '70s, followed by antioxidants, vitamin C, alpha hydroxyl acids, and glycolic acid, to name just a few), and while cosmetics companies want to profit from the existence of these new substances—they're eager to make all the promises about what can be delivered—they aren't prepared to include enough of the active ingredients in their products to make a difference.

The medical community knows that the percentage of active ingredients is critical for the product to be effective. All scientific efficacy studies on cosmetics ingredients have to be reported by naming the exact percentages of the active ingredients. This is because we know that if, for instance, the retinol or the glycolic acid percentage does not reach a certain level, their presence is entirely meaningless from the perspective of performance. It might as well be missing and will do just as much good. If it is present in the right percentages, however, it may irritate some people initially before the product starts to deliver results, which may drive up product returns, the worst fear of cosmetics executives. Also, the right percentages will definitely drive up product price because some of the active ingredients cost in the thousands per kilo.

The skin care companies want to be able to say their products contain the latest, most effective ingredients, but they don't want to face higher product returns and higher production costs. So how do they solve this quandary? With a practice called "angel dusting," manufacturers sprinkle only a little of these powerful ingredients into a jar and call it magic. They are under no legal obligation to reveal the percentages on the label. (Legally, the only time the key ingredient percentage has to be displayed on the label is in the case of sunscreens, acne products, and certain skin faders.) They list the key ingredient on the label without the critical *quantity*, and proclaim that the consumer can hold onto firm skin, smooth out fine lines, and look young forever based on these scientifically based ingredients. In reality, consumers receive little more than gorgeous packaging and expert marketing. Often they do *not* receive the proclaimed ingredients in any meaningful quantities to actually make a difference in the skin. With this listed-on-the-label strategy, major cosmetics companies can charge astounding prices while avoiding the cost and any potential liabilities inherent in using strong ingredients that may cause initial irritation in some people.

So you see, the industry can claim that their products include the scientifically established ingredient and, at the same time, is under *no legal obligation* to give you the ingredients at a percentage where the ingredients actually can exert benefits. From the cosmetics industry's point of view, it's a win/win situation. From your perspective, it is lose/lose.

In addition to the problem of using the right ingredients in the wrong amounts, the major cosmetics houses also rely heavily on creams as the main method of skin-care delivery. Scientists know that creams are not the best media for key ingredient delivery. The reason is: A cream is a good moisturizer, the very particles that make the cream a good moisturizer will, to a large extent, block the way of absorption of those ingredients that are intended to stimulate the skin, perform antioxidant functions, and exfoliate. If the cream is lacking moisturizing capability, it may allow the penetration of key ingredients, which is a great positive; however, this cream will feel dry, irritating, and miserable, which is a huge negative.

The bottom line is that a cream can either feel good, but do very little, or feel miserable, but do everything modern science has to offer. Major cosmetics houses would love for you *not* to understand this concept. This they can sell you a "feel good" cream with minimal amounts of active ingredients, while boasting about the ingredients on the package. They want you to believe what the packaging says and buy a cream that feels good. If it does very little or doesn't work at all it's better for them if you think that it is your skin's fault. That this is just the wrong cream for your skin, and that you need to buy yet another cream.

I remember when I first started my practice, I saw a young woman, Deborah, just barely in her thirties, who came to me because she said she had "problem skin."

"Nothing works for me," Deborah said.

I could see that her pores were very clogged—a sure sign that she had been using heavy creams. So I asked her to bring me the skin products she had used to our next appointment. I will never forget the sight of Deborah arriving for the appointment with a *duffel bag* filled with barely used products. Aside from the waste of money, the bag full of products had eroded Deborah's confidence. She was convinced that she had "problem skin" when in fact the problem was the products.

The greatest fallacy promoted by conventional skin-care companies is that if a product doesn't work, it's your fault.

If you take nothing else from my book, I hope you will realize that your skin is *not* the problem—the problem is the product. If it doesn't work, it is not your fault; take the product back. Nobody can afford to throw away money on useless products.

A great deal can be done to keep your skin from aging. But the first step must be in your mind. Expect results. Realize that it is not your fault if you do not get them. Throw away the fallacies that the skin-care industry has fed you, and let the secrets of science help you keep your skin ageless.

SKIN-CARE FALLACIES

1. <u>FALLACY</u>: **The right cream can solve it all.**

<u>TRUTH</u>: The ultimate jar of cream is a scientific fallacy. If a cream feels good, it may do precious little for your skin because the very moisturizing particles that makes it feel good may block the absorption of the important stimulating ingredients.

Skin care has to be separated into at least two phases:

Phase 1: **Skin-stimulating/building phase,** accomplished with lightweight, quick-absorbing serums that can stimulate the skin's own collagen-building machinery, deliver strong vitamins, and soften the appearance of lines by making the skin thicker and more elastic.

Phase 2: **Skin-sealing phase** or "feel good" moisturizing phase, done by a thick serum or a cream that may help restore the skin lipid barrier and prevents transdermal water loss by sealing the skin.

2. <u>FALLACY</u>: **Skin care that temporarily irritates the skin is bad. Skin care has to feel good all the time.**

<u>TRUTH</u>: To get results in the building phase, the phase that improves the appearance of wrinkles and rejuvenates the skin, you have to use strong ingredients. You may feel a tingle or even see a slight redness. These are signs that the product is working. The skin-sealing phase that immediately follows will make up for the initial tingle and make your skin feel moisturized and comfortable in the next few minutes.

3. <u>FALLACY</u>: **Exfoliation or overexfoliation may thin the skin in the long run.**

<u>TRUTH</u>: This is one of the most crippling fallacies. If you believe this one, you are bound to hinder your own success in anti-aging skin care. Exfoliation actually promotes skin thickness.

This is not an easy concept to understand because it is intuitive to think that the more you wear down and exfoliate the skin, the thinner it becomes. However, this is not how it works in nature.

One of the most important ideas in the science of skin care is that skin is a dynamic organ. The more you wear it down, the more it thickens and grows. Exfoliation stimulates cellular turnover and collagen production, which improves skin thickness. Skin thickness is what ultimately improves the look of lines and wrinkles.

4. FALLACY: The "classic" ingredients of skin care—petrolatum, mineral oils, and waxes, which are still the basics of most skin-care products—work.

TRUTH: Half true. These ingredients work minimally, but they are not the most effective. They do improve the skin lipid barrier somewhat, but these days there are better ingredients that do a far superior job improving the skin lipid barrier using skin identical lipids that are meant for your skin.

I call petrolatum, mineral oils, and waxes "junk food" for your skin—they feel good but they clog your pores. Classic skin care says all you need to do is clean your skin and then moisturize with cream. However, one of the major reasons that your skin may feel dry is that there may be a thick layer of dead skin cells covering the skin, so a moisturizer has a hard time penetrating the skin. The skin should be exfoliated first before moisturizers can work.

5. FALLACY: The major and expensive skin-care brands are using the latest scientific ingredients.

TRUTH: Shockingly, most expensive major cosmetics brands are *not* at the forefront of skin science. They are a few years behind. First they watch the little guys like myself or other doctors' brands introduce new ingredients, and then, once the dust settles, jump in themselves.

They are, after all, large, conservative corporations that move slowly and cautiously. Few of the major companies have medical doctors on staff. It often takes major cosmetics companies years to include a new, effective ingredient—and then they only venture in by using minuscule amounts that may offer minimal benefits. This practice is good for marketing but bad for achieving results.

6. <u>FALLACY:</u> **SPF 15 is adequate protection against the sun.**

TRUTH: Not true. In my opinion, it is far better to use an SPF 30 every day.

I recommend to my patients SPF 30 protection every day, no matter if you are indoors or outdoors and no matter what the season. It is best to use a day cream with a built-in SPF 30 protection instead of a two-step process (first a day cream with *no* protection and then a sunscreen). The reason is that if you have a day cream plus a sunscreen, they will dilute each other on the surface of the skin, and the SPF protection level becomes much less, approximately the average of the two. For instance: If you put on a cream in the morning with an SPF 0, and then you put on foundation with an SPF 8, you will have only approximately SPF 4 protection on your face. Serums do not need to be calculated into this equation because they absorb into the skin.

The sun is the single biggest cause of aging skin. Nearly everything you don't like about your skin comes from exposure to the sun. The sun breaks down the collagen in the skin. If you lose collagen, the skin thins and becomes less elastic. As the skin is pulled by the muscles underneath, it develops wrinkles along the pull lines of the muscles of facial expression. The skin also starts to sag along the jawline. Pores enlarge; enlarged pores begin to fill with sebum and dirt (blackheads). Red capillaries begin to show around the nose, cheeks, and chin because the skin is too thin to cover them properly, and dark skin discolorations (age spots or sun spots) begin to appear. Of course, there's the most dreaded consequences of sun exposure, skin cancer, which is beyond the scope of this book.

The best way to protect your skin is to wear SPF 30 every day, rain or shine. And remember: If you put on a cream in the morning, and then a foundation of SPF 8, you are getting the protection of SPF 4 only.

You do not have to fall victim to the fallacies of skin-care conspiracy. With a little knowledge about the science of skin care, you can fight the effects of aging. In my work, I have taken advantage of the latest developments to create a scientifically proven system that helps your skin look its best. My methods are dramatically different from the conventional approach.

It is never too late to give your skin the attention it deserves—and never too late to educate yourself about the latest innovations in skin care that can help you look younger *now.*

CHAPTER TWO

WHY WE AGE

Carol, a blond, beautiful, moderately overweight forty-six-year-old, came to see me. She had spent a fair amount of time in the sun. She was troubled by ever-increasing lines around her eyes and above her upper lip. Her pores were enlarged, and there were age spots on her cheeks, especially on the side that was exposed to the sun while she was driving her car.

As I examined her, she told me she had been a driven career woman until she was forty. Then she panicked that life was passing her by, and decided to marry and have a child. She was lucky enough to give birth to twins through the miracle of in vitro fertilization, which made her happy beyond her wildest dreams. As we talked, she confided that she finds the stresses of her life overwhelming. Two six-year-olds, an ailing mother who needs daily care, her job—it had all become too much. She did not have the energy, the focus, the memory, and the physical stamina she needed to handle all of her responsibilities.

"I don't recognize myself anymore," Carol told me with tears in her eyes. "I don't look like me. I don't feel like me."

Carol's problem is one I see all the time: Middle age had begun for her, and it had come as one of the busiest and most-demanding stages of her life.

WHEN MIDDLE AGE ARRIVES

At what age does middle age set in? I can't give you a single number that defines the beginning of middle age because it is so variable for each of us. But, unfortunately, when it happens, you can't miss it; you don't have to look for subtleties. You would hope that it would happen gradually, but for most of us the change is quite sudden. One day, you just feel it.

One of the first things you notice is that your energy level is not the same as it used to be. You tire more easily climbing stairs. You cannot walk as fast. You feel as if you need more sleep, so you go to bed earlier, only to find that the extra sleep does not help your tiredness very much. Sleep is less restful. You wake up earlier and feel tired; you just cannot shake the constant lack of energy.

The skin begins to thin. Lines start to show around the eyes and above the lips. The chin loses definition. The lips thin and wrinkle. Age spots appear. Hair loses its luster, shine, flexibility, and turns dry and brittle, and we lose it, lots of it.

Then there is the change in mental capacities. Your memory is not what it used to be. Learning ability, concentration, and mental stamina all decline. It now takes many repetitions to learn a foreign word. It is difficult to stay up all night, when it was once so easy. Jet lag may be more of a problem.

And, of course, the fat begins to settle around the middle—in the abdomen for men, and in the abdomen and hips for women. The waistline thickens, and what you eat, or don't eat, makes little difference. You feel you eat much less, yet the middle section just keeps thickening. You feel as if weight comes on just by thinking about food, and it never seems to come off.

Sex may be less enjoyable, and in general, the ability to feel alive, to experience joy, pleasure, and passion does not come as easily as it used to. The confidence of a winner and the sense of indestructibility may have evaporated. The feeling of well-being for no particular reason may now be rare or nonexistent. You might think this is because you have so much more to worry about now than you used to, but that is not the reason. The reason is physiological; it is inherent in the aging process, in the changes of the human body and brain chemistry.

A slight depression sometimes sets in, or at least a case of the blues. It is no longer easy to feel excitement—it takes a lot more stimulation to feel a lot less joy. So you may settle for a more steady and even, but a far less joyful, existence.

But you don't have to settle. Fortunately, this is a time in history when you can postpone the look and feel of middle age. Modern science has shown that with lifestyle and dietary changes, with the right supplements and skin-care ingredients, you can stay younger—and look more youthful—longer than was ever imagined before.

THE THEORIES OF HOW WE AGE

Scientists have identified several possible mechanisms of aging—a set of theories with technical names that describe the wear and tear on our cells that constitute aging. Each mechanism plays a role in growing older. They are not mutually exclusive, but they coexist. In fact, each theory provides an explanation of the same preprogrammed process called aging, simply seen from a different point of view. This always reminds me of the tiny Lilliputians in *Gulliver's Travels* who each have a different description of "the giant" who arrived in their midst. They were all correct, but the differences in their descriptions was in the angle at which they saw "the giant."

Why is it necessary to understand these theories of aging? Why are they important in a book about skin care? Because the only way we can combat the reasons we age is by understanding them first. When we can see the whole, complex process at work, we can keep "the giant" from overwhelming us. So let's take a brief look at each theory.

THE FREE-RADICAL OR OXIDATIVE THEORY OF AGING

This theory was first advanced by Denham Harman, M.D., Ph.D., in 1956. Free radicals are molecules that have lost an electron in their interaction with other molecules. Consequently, they become unstable and reactive, and begin searching for a "mate" that will provide the missing component. A free radical molecule will attach to any healthy molecule, in a destructive manner, to complete itself. It will steal an electron from a healthy molecule, rendering the donor molecule dysfunctional. Over time, this chain reaction will translate into wrinkles, gray hair, thinning skin, and weaker muscles, in addition to compromised liver and kidney functions, and all other signs of aging. We take antioxidants (nutrients that are found in vitamins, amino acids, and other natural substances) to try to counteract this deadly chain of events.

Some of the most important dietary antioxidants to combat the problem are beta-carotene, vitamin C, grapeseed extract, selenium, carnosine, vitamin E, alpha lipoic acid, resveratrol from grapes, CoQ10, and melatonin. A comprehensive collection of these ingredients should be part of your overall anti-aging plan. (In chapter 3, I will discuss supplements in more detail.)

THE MEMBRANE THEORY OF AGING

First proposed by a Hungarian scientist, Imre S. Nagy, this theory states that cell membranes become less pliable as we grow older, due to the loss of lipid and water stored within each cell. This loss impedes the efficiency of the flow of fluids in and out of the cells, which can lead to toxic accumulations of cellular material, known as lipofuscin. As we age, lipofuscin deposits become more and more present in the brain, heart, lungs, skin, and everywhere else throughout the body. Age spots can be composed of lipofuscin. The best supplements to combat the problem are hyaluronic acid, acetyl-l-carnitine, and carnosine.

THE MITOCHONDRIAL THEORY OF AGING

Mitochondria are tiny power plants in every cell of the body that supply energy. Cells cannot borrow energy from each other; therefore, if the mitochondria of a particular cell fail, so does the cell. Enhancing and protecting mitochondria is an essential part of combating the effects of aging. The best supplements to attack the problem are pregnenolone and acetyl-l-carnitine, in addition to the antioxidants previously mentioned.

THE GLYCATION AND PROTEIN CARBONYLATION THEORY OF AGING

Glycation may be the single most important reason why we age. Under normal conditions, glucose is inside the cells, being utilized as fuel for energy. But when glycation occurs, glucose attaches to proteins or to DNA. With the attachment of glucose, the function of the protein and DNA becomes irreversibly compromised.

The problem begins when the circulating glucose level in the blood is high. This is the time when most glycation takes place. Therefore, keeping our blood glucose levels as low as possible is an important goal from an anti-aging perspective. Fortunately, there is a lot we can do toward this end. Keeping our glucose and carbohydrate consumption in check is one of the most important efforts we can make to combat the effects of aging. Carnosine is a helpful dietary supplement that helps reduce glycation.

Protein carbonylation is a related process in which a carbonyl group attaches to a protein, destroying its function. Carnosine is a key player in protecting the protein from carbonylation as well.

THE TELOMERES THEORY OF AGING

Telomeres (the sequences of nucleic acids extending from the ends of chromosomes) shorten every time a cell divides, which is believed to lead to cellular damage. Each time a cell divides, it duplicates itself a little less perfectly than the time before, and this eventually leads to cellular dysfunction and aging. In the future, there may be a way to introduce an enzyme into the cell that may protect the telomere; but for now, there is not much we can do. Instead, we can pursue other anti-aging strategies where we can actually make a difference.

THE HORMONAL THEORY OF AGING

This theory states that as we age, our delicate hormonal feedback mechanism breaks down and nearly all our hormonal levels decline rather dramatically—all our *beneficial* hormones, that is. Levels of hormones such as human growth hormone (HGH), estrogen, progesterone, testosterone, DHEA, pregnenolone, thyroid hormone, melatonin, and thymus decline.

Unfortunately, a few "dark," pro-aging hormones increase as we age. The key one is insulin, and I will elaborate on this later. Cortisol levels also go up. Cortisol is associated with stress states and is responsible for muscle breakdown, uncontrollable midsection weight gain, and thinning of the skin. Prolactin is another "dark" hormone that rises with the years and helps us to put on fat.

According to the hormonal theory of aging, nearly all hormones decline with age. One of the keys to anti-aging success is a broad-range, comprehensive approach to replace all the missing hormones. I will give you my suggestions for counteracting these hormonal changes in chapter 8.

THE METABOLIC THEORY OF AGING

All of the above theories describe and explain the aging process from different perspectives. However, they are not mutually exclusive; they work together to describe the extremely complex process we call aging.

In my anti-aging work, I have found it most useful to focus on what I refer to as the metabolic theory of aging. This theory spotlights the effects of the giant of the pro-aging dark hormones: insulin. Insulin, often termed the master hormone of metabolism, increases dramatically with age—less in some, more in others. I think it is critical to understand how insulin works, does its damage, and how we can control its pro-aging influence. Through diet, we can have a profound effect on this metabolic giant.

THE MASTER HORMONE OF METABOLISM: INSULIN

Almost everyone is familiar with insulin as the regulator of blood sugar, and indeed this is its main function. Without insulin we would die within days, if not hours. However, too much insulin in the blood has profound pro-aging effects.

The problem begins if insulin levels go abnormally high during the course of the day. When glucose enters the bloodstream, insulin is secreted from the pancreas within approximately three to five minutes. The function of insulin is to usher the glucose out of your blood as quickly as possible and into your cells, where it is used as fuel. Each cell has receptors for insulin, much like trapdoors, through which the hormone enters. As we age, we lose more and more of these trapdoors; we have fewer and fewer insulin receptors on cells. This means that we need to produce more and more insulin to find the fewer and fewer entryways into the cells. Remember, the goal is to get the glucose into the cells and out of the blood as quickly as possible. In medical terms, as we age, we become more and more insulin-resistant.

When you were a child, and all your insulin receptors were functioning perfectly, your glucose metabolism worked flawlessly. If you ate a dish of ice cream, a little bit of insulin was secreted to clear the sugar from your blood; then your insulin levels returned to normal almost immediately. When you are a middle-aged adult, things are a lot less rosy. The same amount of ice cream may trigger a lot more insulin. Why? Because there are fewer trapdoors (insulin receptors), so a lot more insulin is necessary to find the fewer receptors. This means that there is more insulin in your blood for longer periods of time.

So what is the big deal? you may ask. More insulin in the blood for longer time periods: how bad could that be?

Very, very bad. Insulin (and hyperinsulinemia, a chronically elevated insulin level) is the enemy of youth and health. During the times when your insulin level is high, your body is adding fat onto your waistline and raising your blood pressure. Insulin also increases triglycerides, the tiny particles that comprise your body fat and are predictive of heart disease. And excess insulin makes you tired all the time, in part because your cells aren't getting all the fuel they need. Insulin makes the kidneys retain salt and fluids, further elevating your blood pressure. Insulin takes an active role in thickening and hardening your arterial walls, a condition that is the precursor for heart disease and poor peripheral circulation. Poor peripheral circulation is one of the fastest ways to a decline of the elasticity, resilience, and radiance of your skin.

Then, to top it all off, insulin's extended presence makes it nearly impossible to take off fat. As long as your insulin levels are consistently elevated, the effects will override even your best dieting efforts. Whenever you eat some carbohydrates, your body has to call in an army of insulin to do a small cleanup job quickly because of the lack of receptor sites. And the army of insulin will linger in the blood a lot longer than a small battalion. As time goes by, blood sugar rises higher and stays up longer after a carbohydrate meal because the insulin can no longer do a good cleanup job. So the body makes *even more* insulin. A high level of glucose in the blood causes glycation, one of the main reasons why we age. Glycation, as you recall, is the binding of sugar to proteins that compromises the proteins' enzymatic function, destroys DNA, and promotes aging.

High levels of insulin also activate your cholesterol-making machinery. You may think that a six-ounce porterhouse steak will send your cholesterol soaring, but in fact, the consumption of red meat has a minuscule effect on your cholesterol levels compared to what an even moderately elevated insulin level can do. The cholesterol you eat is responsible for only 20 to 30 percent of your circulating cholesterol levels; the rest is manufactured courtesy of insulin. It may seem counterintuitive at first, but eating carbohydrates, even complex carbohydrates, has more impact on your cholesterol levels than ingesting high-fat foods. Yet still, some leading nutrition authorities recommend a low-fat, high-complex carbohydrate diet for individuals with high cholesterol—exactly what may send their cholesterol levels sky high.

As we age, glucose metabolism becomes compromised for much of the population. Many of us actually become slightly diabetic. Don't panic. Diabetes is a frightening word, and I'm not suggesting that you're suffering from a serious, chronic illness. Most of us never reach the level of carbohydrate metabolism dysfunction that can be clinically diagnosed as diabetes, but we may spend most of our adult life hovering on the border, with a condition called subclinical diabetes.

There is no doubt that these insulin-related metabolic changes foster aging. For me, in fact, they define the root of aging and the root of the major degenerative changes such as obesity, heart disease, type 2 diabetes, senile dementia of vascular origin (the most prevalent form), and senescent mental decline.

Insulin is so important from an anti-aging perspective, I will venture to say that insulin resistance is perhaps one of the key metabolic reasons why we age—hence my proposal of the metabolic theory of aging.

However, everything in nature has its opposite, and we have been given a balancing hormone for insulin. It's called glucagon. Glucagon works in ways that are exactly counter to insulin. It shifts the metabolism from a fat-depositing mode into a fat-burning mode. It decreases the body's production of cholesterol. It prompts the kidneys to release fluids. And it helps to regress arterial thickening.

The problem is that while large amounts of insulin are flooding your system, glucagon can't get a word in edgewise. During most of the hours of the day, glucagon is totally outnumbered and dominated by insulin. Insulin runs the metabolic machinery most of the hours of the day, busily making us put on weight while glucagon is waiting in the background for the few hours at night when the insulin level is sufficiently down, so it can run the metabolic show for a while.

What is the solution? The key is to keep your insulin levels at bay for as many hours of the day as possible. You would achieve that by consuming the absolute minimum of carbohydrates, avoiding simple sugars, so as not to wake up insulin.

Suppose you have a meal of proteins and fats only. As far as insulin is concerned, this is a nonevent. Nothing happened. It will not even bother to come out of its cage in the pancreas. So you bought yourself a few baseline low-insulin hours (insulin is never at zero) without feeling hungry. On the other hand, if you had bread with your meal, or a sugary dessert, insulin would be all over your blood, churning out cholesterol, triglycerides, increasing your blood pressure, and putting fat around your waistline for the next three to five hours, or longer.

Insulin, in the right amounts, is life-sustaining. But too much of it is disastrous. And unfortunately, as we grow older, its level rises for nearly all of us.

Is the insulin story applicable to you? You can find out by looking at the questionnaire on page 29 in the next chapter. It will help you determine if you are insulin-resistant. The chances are that unless you are perfectly thin and able to eat as much as you want, whenever you want, you are not an exception to the rule.

HGH: THE MASTER YOUTH HORMONE

Have you ever wondered why some middle-aged celebrities don't look anything like the rest of us? Their posture, their trim, muscular figures, the way they move, all convey energy. And their lineless faces, thick hair, and strong voices belie their years. What do they know that most people do not? What do they do?

Well, they have access and money to pay for the best that anti-aging medicine has to offer. I ought to know because many of them come to me, arriving at my office in black limousines with tinted windows, surrounded by security guards and personal assistants. Many of them come to me to receive injections of human growth hormone (HGH). They find that it makes their voices stronger and younger, gives them a remarkable edge in the battle of muscle versus fat, restores energy, sharpens memory (great for learning the lines), lessens depression and anxiety, thickens hair, and tightens the face. Need I say more?

They do not have to ask how much it costs. The rest of us do (about $1,000 to $1,500 per month). Now, if it is not in your budget to remain youthful with this easy and expensive way, take heart, because I am going to tell you exactly how you can achieve similar results in a much more inexpensive way—with my diet and supplement plan.

What exactly is HGH, and how does it hold so much power?

As its name suggests, human growth hormone is the hormone that helps your body grow, maintain, and repair itself. It's secreted by the pituitary gland at night and is a major player in your metabolism, integral to every aspect of your body's ability to burn calories, use energy, and eliminate waste. While all the other major pituitary hormones affect a principal target gland (such as the thyroid gland, adrenal cortex, ovaries, and testicles), HGH, in contrast, affects virtually *all* tissues of the body. HGH is a profound anabolic, tissue-building, and tissue-repairing entity that increases the rate of protein synthesis in every cell of the body. It mobilizes fat from fat deposits; uses fat for energy; and is, perhaps, the most important fat-burning mechanism ever identified.

HGH appears to hold a key function in the process of aging. Its benefits are so significant, it is often called the master hormone of youth. It has been suggested that many of the signs of aging (such as decreased energy; loss of stamina, muscle strength, and muscle tone; increased abdominal fat; wrinkles; thinning hair; decline in sexual and immune functions and memory; bone fragility; and poor sleep) can be attributed, to some extent, to the age-associated loss of HGH.

When you're young, you have HGH in abundance. It peaks during adolescence, then drops dramatically at about age thirty-five, continuing to drop at a rate of about 15 percent per decade. By ages forty-five to fifty, most people have already reached "elderly" levels of growth hormone production. By age sixty-five you're making only 25 percent of what you made when you were a young adult.

Until 1990 we did not know much about HGH, except that children who are extremely short can grow to near-normal or normal height with additional HGH, which, of course, is a remarkable benefit. However, until recently there was little research on the effects of HGH on adults.

The groundbreaking study elucidating the role of HGH in aging was conducted at the Medical College of Wisconsin by Dr. Daniel Rudman and published in the *New England Journal of Medicine* in 1990. Dr. Rudman treated twelve men, aged sixty-one to eighty-one, with a three-times-a-week injected dose of recombinant HGH. Six months later, at the study's conclusion, the men had lost 14.4 percent of body fat (mostly from the abdomen); gained 8.8 percent in lean body mass (mostly muscle); increased bone density of the spine by 1.6 percent; and regenerated 19 percent of their liver and 17 percent of their spleen; and thickened their skin by 7.1 percent, resulting in fewer wrinkles.

"The effects," Dr. Rudman reported, "were the equivalent in magnitude to the changes incurred during ten to twenty years of aging."

The Rudman study opened the floodgates to hundreds of subsequent studies of HGH and aging, and the findings have been remarkably consistent. The administration of HGH has been shown to increase energy, cardiac muscle strength, lung capacity, kidney function, memory, concentration, and sexual performance. It also enhances immune function; improves skin, hair, and nails; encourages deeper, more restful sleep; and dramatically lifts the mood and sense of well-being—results that make it very clear why all of us should be trying to optimize our HGH levels.

The most reliable way to increase HGH is through injections, but, admittedly, that's not for everyone. HGH treatments are prohibitively expensive and must be done under strict medical supervision. Don't even think about buying HGH injections on the Internet or at your gym! The dosages must be based on your weight and blood levels, and careful monitoring is essential.

Even though the scientific findings on HGH have been extremely positive so far, the jury hasn't come back with a definitive verdict. If you read the papers and watch the TV news, you may have heard some negative reports about HGH. It is true that HGH can produce some real, worrisome side effects, including water retention, increased blood pressure, and carpal tunnel syndrome. But all of these are a result of overdosing, and once the dosage is cut back, the problems resolve themselves. Then the treatment can continue at a lesser dosage. The only way to overdose on HGH would be to ignore and override your doctor's instructions.

The benefits of HGH administration are truly remarkable—life-changing, in many instances. My patients report improvement in energy, stamina, mental focus, and memory. Their learning ability and concentration greatly improve, and they tell me that they sleep more deeply and wake up more fully rested. Please note that these descriptions of patient experiences are not just coming from my practice. These are scientifically studied and documented. Of course, individual results may vary. However, in my clinical experience, I have seen nothing that can even come close to the impact of HGH.

BUYER BEWARE

You may have seen one of the countless promotions for amino acid stimulants for Human Growth Hormone (HGH). These products claim that certain combinations and quantities of amino acids can trigger the release of already manufactured HGH from the pituitary gland, thereby increasing this master hormone of youth. This just makes me wince. These companies take the genuine, proven results of medical, injectable HGH replacement and imply that the same benefits can be obtained from oral amino-acid-releasing HGH powders. I want you to know that these claims are a far cry from the truth. The benefits derived from genuine, injectable HGH hormone replacement are much greater than any benefits that come from these powders or pills. So you really should take these claims with a grain of salt.

These supplements are based on the scientific fact that as we grow older, our production of HGH in the pituitary gland declines, and much of what we attribute to the effects of aging is the effect of a decrease in the level of HGH. But these amino acid releasers won't significantly increase our HGH level. First, many of the products are ineffective because they simply contain insufficient amounts of the right amino acid components. But no matter how effective an AA releaser might be initially, it won't stay effective for long because after sixty to ninety days, the level of HGH stored in the pituitary is exhausted. At this point, all amino acid releasers will stop working because there is no HGH supply left to be released. Time must pass for the HGH level to regenerate. The bottom line is that you should take these anti-aging claims with caution and listen to your body's response.

However, I couldn't possibly recommend injections for everyone. Each case must be decided independently, between patient and doctor.

As I've said, there is a great deal we can do to imitate many of the benefits of HGH injections. As one of my patients put it, we can use "the difficult but inexpensive way." It takes more work, but you can get great results without injecting anything into your system.

It begins with dietary changes, which, I admit, are somewhat difficult. Yet, if you follow through, the rewards can be remarkable. Your diet is the biological underpinning of your anti-aging plan.

THE MATTER OF WEIGHT

Obesity is one of the most serious pro-aging factors. Carrying excess pounds increases the risk of heart attack, stroke, other serious cardiovascular and respiratory problems, certain cancers, high cholesterol, gallstones, and diabetes. The more you weigh, the greater the danger. *Obesity also severely decreases your natural level of HGH.* Studies have shown that being even moderately overweight reduces your HGH levels well below the measure that your age might justify. Low HGH levels make you burn even less fat, make you even more tired, sluggish, and unable to build muscle, sleep less well, perpetuate the weight, and age you before your time. *But—here's the good news—any weight loss soon leads to a substantial rise in the level of HGH.*

So you need to do your very best to lose excess weight you may be carrying. Studies have found that even moderate overweight status will significantly lower your HGH levels. On the other hand, even moderate weight loss will lead to a substantial HGH level increase, which can translate into a clearly perceivable and very pleasant experience that will encourage you to lose even more weight. One of the joys of losing a significant amount of weight is a surge of your formerly suppressed HGH levels. This translates into a happier outlook and an improved sense of well-being. These feelings can be easily attributed to losing weight; however, HGH is the most likely mediator in the chain of events.

THE BATTLE OF THE HORMONES

As I explained earlier, one of the serious consequences of eating a diet high in refined sugar and other carbohydrates has to do with insulin. In midlife, many of us (perhaps most of us) lose some of the insulin receptor sites on our cells, as well as the sensitive feedback mechanism that regulates the insulin and glucose connection, and develop some insulin resistance. These in turn cause a perpetually elevated insulin level throughout much of the day, with all the concomitant damage. Insulin also inhibits the release of HGH, which is another critical piece of the puzzle. So, in addition to all the pro-aging influence of insulin, it undermines the activity of the most important anti-aging hormone of all.

Based on scientific evidence, aging, to a large extent, can be viewed as a conflict between the powerful *pro-aging* hormone insulin, the master hormone of metabolism, and the equally powerful *anti-aging* human growth hormone, the master hormone of youth.

The winner in this war can be determined by your diet. If you think of insulin as the sleeping foe who you don't wish to awaken, you can aid HGH by *not* eating too many carbohydrates. They can then become your most powerful allies in avoiding premature aging.

In the next chapter I will show you how to create a diet that will help you maintain your ideal weight, enhance your complexion, and keep the years from showing. By the time you finish, you'll have a good idea of how much premature aging can be avoided through the choices you make—not only of *what* you eat, but also *when* you eat.

CHAPTER THREE

Dr. Denese's Anti-Aging Diet and Supplement Plan

As youngsters, we could eat as much as we wanted and not gain an ounce. As we age, of course, this changes dramatically. We eat much less now than we used to, yet still gain weight. And when we try to lose the weight, we run into remarkable resistance. We starve ourselves, cut our portions down to a size that is barely enough to feed a cat, yet we still lose the battle of the bulge. Why?

Remember in the previous chapter that we talked about aging as the battle between the pro-aging hormone insulin and the anti-aging human growth hormone? We explained that many of us become more and more insulin-resistant with age, resulting in faulty carbohydrate metabolism, which makes it very hard for us to control our weight. Furthermore, excess insulin may inhibit the release of human growth hormone, so we lose out on some of the anti-aging benefits that human growth hormone can provide. But the good news is that there are some scientifically based dietary rules that may allow you to gain control over insulin resistance. Let us see first, however, if you are, like about 40 percent of the U.S. adult population, slightly insulin-resistant. Consider the following statements. How many apply to you?

- I gain weight easily.

- The older I get, the harder it is to lose weight.

- Most of my excess weight is in my midsection, stomach, and hips.

- I often crave bread, chips, crackers, and other crunchy snacks.

- I rarely crave cheese, chicken, or other meats.

- I love pasta and baked goods.

- When I eat cookies, chocolate, or pastries, it's difficult for me to stop.

- I find sweets and chocolate comforting.

- A meal doesn't feel complete without dessert.

- I must eat as soon as I get up in the morning.

- I need to eat lunch as early as I can; I'm never able to postpone lunch until the middle of the afternoon.

- I'm usually hungry within two hours after a meal.

- Hunger affects my moods; I become irritated and tense.

- If I go too long without eating, my mind becomes cloudy and I have difficulty focusing.

- High-protein, low-carbohydrate diets have worked for me, but I missed carbohydrates terribly.

If you answered "not applicable" to most of these statements, then you are either very young or very lucky, and you are definitely in the minority. Most adults suffer from some carbohydrate metabolism deficiency. In fact, I see this condition in 40 percent of my patients over age forty-five. Please understand that this does not mean you are diabetic. It means that you are what doctors call subclinically insulin-resistant.

Personally, I answered, "yes" to every statement. I am the perfect example of someone who is subclinically diabetic. My fiancé calls me an aspiring diabetic, which makes me laugh every time.

If I were to eat a diet high in carbohydrates, I would be as wide as I am tall. When I eat carbohydrates, my insulin level goes sky high and stays there for hours. When I avoid carbs, I feel great and my weight remains exactly where I like it.

In this chapter I want to share with you my anti-aging diet plan, a plan that I use myself with success. It starts with knowing not only what to eat, but also when to eat it.

THE ANTI-AGING DIET PLAN

BEGIN YOUR EATING PLAN AT NIGHT

The best thing you can do to start out your anti-aging diet program is to go to bed with no carbohydrates in your system. If you eat no carbs for at least three hours before you go to sleep, you will build a good foundation for the next day.

STARTING THE DAY: BREAKFAST

In the morning, your metabolic goal is to not wake up your insulin for as long as possible. When insulin wakes, so does your appetite and your tendency to add fat to your middle. The way to keep insulin asleep is to start the day with protein. There is one more key step to take: ingest a large dose (about 3000 mg) of essential fatty acids, a long chain Omega 3 from fish oil, for reasons that I will elaborate on later.

As you recall, human growth hormone (HGH), with all its re-markable anti-aging benefits, is released by the pituitary gland when you reach the deep stage of sleep. If you eat carbs before going to bed, then you produce fresh insulin, in addition to your baseline insulin. The insulin may remain high in your system long enough to coincide with the release of HGH, inhibiting the release of HGH to a lesser or greater extent, thus depriving you of the benefits of HGH for the next day. As you know, HGH may help you to sleep deeper, burn more fat while asleep, and wake up with more energy in the morning. Carbs at night with the concomitant insulin re-lease may deprive you of some of these benefits.

As long as your insulin hormone is dormant, your glucagon hor-mone rules. Glucagon is your friend because its effect is the exact oppo-site of insulin's: it breaks down fat, keeps your appetite depressed, and keeps your blood pressure down and cholesterol levels low. The way to keep your insulin dormant is by not feeding it any carbohydrates.

It is critical that you start the day without any carbohydrates. It is more important than at any other time of the day—first, because in-sulin responds much more briskly in the morning, and second, because you have the entire day ahead of you. If you get into an insulin-driven mode early, you will be hungry and you will likely be gaining weight instead of losing or maintaining weight that day. Eat only protein in the morning, take an essential fatty acid supplement, and stay on a low-carb diet during the day for as long as you can manage. If you can make it carb-free until lunch, you're off and running. If you are not actively trying to lose weight, but you are in a maintenance mode, you can have some low-glycemic-index fruits, preferably berries, in the morning.

Coffee is problematic, I'm sorry to say. It releases glucose from in-ternal sources that can trigger insulin, even if you curb the carbs. So it's best to avoid it. Unfortunately, tea is not a good alternative, because the problem is the presence of caffeine, not coffee per se, and tea also contains caffeine. While tea has many beneficial antioxidant properties, if you suffer from faulty glucose metabolism and have a tendency to gain weight, you may need to strike a balance with your tea intake as well. Decaffeinated coffee or tea or, better yet, herbal tea may be a better choice.

You will find that keeping your blood sugar levels stable in the morning by avoiding carbs will help you fight midday fatigue, hunger, and carb cravings. Other benefits include an increased ability to concentrate and a better sense of well-being than usual. Give it a try.

Personally, if I eat only proteins in the morning, no carbohydrates at all—not a bite of toast, a drop of orange juice, and certainly no potatoes or cereal (not even high-fiber cereal)—I do not have the usual midday, "I could faint from hunger" feeling by noon. I can wait for lunch until two, and I find I have minimal appetite for the rest of the day. On the other hand, if I start the day with carbohydrates, I'm tired and terribly hungry by noon and continue to crave carbs and remain hungry all day long. I know that starting the day with fish, steak, chicken, or eggs and no freshly baked rolls, jam, orange juice, cereal, and the like is not fun. I do not like it either, but the payoff is worth it. With no carbs, you buy yourself a fresh mind, no food cravings, minimal appetite, no midday tiredness, and a good handle on your weight. As an adult and especially if you have, like me, a tendency for weight gain, a classic breakfast of freshly baked rolls, honey, preservatives, cereal (even if it is high in fiber), orange juice, and coffee should be a rare luxury. The price tag is just too high for every day.

THE MIDDAY MEAL: LUNCH

I have always envied people who can be casual about when they eat lunch. Until I began refraining from all carbohydrates at breakfast, I simply had to eat by noon or my brain would shut down. Now I can go without lunch until two o'clock. I cannot tell you how impossible this would be for me if I had even a glass of orange juice in the morning.

Try to hold out for as long as you can without carbs during the day; it will put you ahead in the game. When you are ready to eat lunch, choose protein (ideally fish), green salads, and low-starch vegetables.

Unrefined carbohydrates from fruits and vegetables release their sugars more slowly. How slowly depends on the food. The effect of each food on your glucose and insulin levels is quantified by a system called the Glycemic Index. The lower a food falls in this index, the better it is for purposes of this diet. (See the chart on pages 36–37.)

I recommend that you take the largest portion of your daily dose of vitamin supplements at lunch, since it is better to take vitamins and other supplements with a full meal. (See pages 37–50 for detailed information about the supplements I recommend.)

If you've lasted until lunch without carbohydrates and were able to control your carbohydrate intake at lunch, insulin hasn't had a chance to settle more fat on your middle. In fact, you burned fat with glucagon. In addition, insulin wasn't around to raise your blood pressure and make more cholesterol. You've exposed yourself for many continuous hours to the magic of glucagon. You're in a win/win situation, and you'll feel the benefits immediately.

THE LATE-AFTERNOON BREAK: SNACK TIME

By the middle of the afternoon, almost everyone experiences a slump. If you've worked in an office, you've probably noticed the phenomenon among your colleagues of the late-afternoon rush for coffee and something sweet to provide a pick-me-up.

By this time of the day you can afford to have a snack that contains carbohydrates. Fruit is a good choice. But avoid pastries, cookies, or sugar and flour snacks of any kind. Again, fruits that are low on the Glycemic Index are the most beneficial for you at this point.

YOU NEED WATER . . .

Drink about half a gallon of water a day. It's a large amount, but that's our daily requirement. It's essential for beautiful skin, of course. It's also important for renal function and blood circulation.

Whenever you feel tired, ask yourself: "Am I dehydrated?" Your first response should be to drink half a quart of water or more. Frequently, the primary reason for feeling tired is lack of hydration. It is easily reversible. Don't overlook the benefits of water as a pick-me-up before you reach for coffee or another stimulant.

THE LAST MEAL: DINNER

For dinner, try to eat more protein, low-starch vegetables, and some low-glycemic fruits. No bread, pasta, or potatoes; leave them for the kids, who can still eat them without gaining weight. Take the rest of your supplements at dinner. Make sure to finish your meal at least three hours before you go to bed. Do not eat any carbs three hours before bedtime or you will wake up your insulin and prevent HGH from doing its good work while you sleep.

HOW WOULD YOU LIKE THAT PREPARED?

When you hear this question and you think about ordering (or cooking) your meat rare, medium rare, or well done, remember: foods cooked at very high temperatures are more likely to contain toxins. This includes foods that are fried, barbecued, broiled, and even cooked in the microwave. While overcooked animal products are the worst offenders, extreme heat can scorch the natural sugars in any food and create toxins. You can reduce exposure to toxins by eating foods that are steamed, boiled, poached, stewed, stir-fried, or cooked in a slow cooker. Such methods not only cook at lower temperatures, they also preserve more valuable nutrients. Finally, eating more low–Glycemic Index fresh fruits and raw and steamed vegetables has great antioxidant and thus anti-aging benefits.

MAKING FOOD CHOICES

FOODS TO ENJOY

Egg whites are an excellent staple in your diet because they contain the highest usable form of protein for humans. Egg white omelets are my favorite breakfast choice. Try to avoid consuming egg yolks, however, because of the cholesterol and arachidonic acid (AA), an unfavorable fat type.

Cottage cheese and yogurt (sugar-free), in moderation, are good choices to help you meet your need for calcium. There are a few low-carb yogurts on the market today that can fit well into your diet.

Whole milk is more filling than the low-fat alternatives because of its fat content. In addition, it triggers less of an insulin reaction than its reduced-fat counterpart.

Choose fresh whole fruits over fruit juices. In fact, leave fruit juices to the kids. Whole fruits are a rich source of fiber, vitamins, and, importantly, will make you feel more full than juice. The amount of nutrients in juices is minimal, especially if they have been sitting on a shelf for a long time, and the damage they can do in terms of insulin reaction is so vast that it's just not a fair trade.

I especially recommend berries of all kinds. They taste delicious, are full of minerals, are high in antioxidants, and are low on the Glycemic Index.

Dress your salads with vinegar and oil. Be careful of commercial dressings; many of them are loaded with carbohydrates. Read the labels and avoid any dressing that contains more than three or four grams of carbs per tablespoon.

Nuts and seeds have nearly zero carbohydrates, and they won't trigger an insulin reaction. They're also high in nutrients.

Whole-grain breads can be permitted on this diet—however, only in minimal amounts and only in the afternoon. Try to eat bread in isolation from protein. Wait about two to three hours after eating bread before you eat any protein. In this way, the insulin reaction to bread will not be made even more costly with the extra calories and fat from protein.

FOODS TO AVOID

Sweet baked goods, cakes, cookies, bagels, muffins, scones, and sweet cereals are all out of the question.

Beans, lentils, and other legumes are very fattening for anyone who is even moderately insulin-resistant.

White bread, white rice, pasta, and oatmeal should all be eliminated from your diet as well.

High Glycemic Index fruits such as bananas, and even some sweet apples are also on the prohibited list.

THE SMART CHOICE GUIDE

Selecting foods that will help to keep your insulin levels low isn't difficult once you know what to look for. Here are a few lists to help you put together nutritious, antioxidant-rich meals.

Foods Low on the Glycemic Index:

Asparagus	Cantaloupe
Cabbage	Citrus fruits

Honeydew melon   Pears
Kiwi fruit   Raspberries
Leafy greens   Zucchini
Peaches

Foods high on the Glycemic Index:

Bananas   Pancakes
Breads   Papaya
Carrots   Pasta
Cereals   Potatoes
Corn   Rice
Fruit juices   Waffles
Mangoes

THE TOP TEN ANTI-AGING FOODS

According to USDA researchers, the best fruits and vegetables that act as antioxidants are:

Beets   Oranges
Blueberries   Plums
Broccoli   Red grapes
Brussels sprouts   Spinach
Kale   Strawberries

DR. DENESE'S GUIDE TO SUPPLEMENTS

In addition to eating the right foods at the right time, we can boost our anti-aging abilities by the addition of the right diet supplements. When you fuel your body with healthy supplements, you obtain energy, growth, and renewal. Here are the supplements I recommend. Let's start with the basics.

FIBER

Fiber is remarkably important: It detoxifies the bowels and facilitates normal stool elimination. Yet the truth is that nearly all of us are chronically fiber-deficient.

Today, the problem of constipation is much more widespread than is generally realized. Constipation in adults is almost invariably caused by the lack of sufficient fiber in the diet. But it is not your fault. If you ate enough to have sufficient fiber in your system, you would need to eat so much that you would grow fat. Ideally, we need about forty grams of fiber a day. This is a remarkably high number, considering that a good-sized salad contains about five to six grams, an apple two to three grams, and proteins almost no grams. It is exceedingly difficult to eat enough fiber. It's quite a dilemma. If you're on a low-carb, high-protein diet, then you simply cannot eat enough coarse, high-fiber bread and unrefined rice and fruits to supply the fiber you need. So you really have no choice but to take supplemental fiber, and to take it in very generous quantities. I recommend Metamucil or Citrucel (the sugar-free, powder varieties) every day. You get much more fiber from a few tablespoonfuls of diluted powder than from a few tablets. You may find that you want to take even more than what the bottle suggests, and certainly not less. Continue increasing your dosage until you're taking enough to avoid any problems with your bowel movements. As long as you are still experiencing any constipation, you are not taking enough. Take as much as you need for the problem to go away. It will seem like a lot of fiber—well, it will be a lot of fiber—but what can you do? It is better than the alternative. I do not think that taking laxatives habitually is a good idea at all. Why take a drug to solve a perfectly natural problem, especially when there is a perfectly natural solution to it?

A word of caution: Do not take fiber with your vitamins. It can coat vitamins and interfere with their absorption. Take your vitamins with your meals. Vitamins on an empty stomach often cause nausea. Fiber is best taken before meals because it may contribute to a sense of fullness in your stomach so you eat less.

MULTIVITAMINS AND MINERALS

Supplemental vitamins and nutrients are necessary for a simple reason: you cannot consume sufficient vitamins and minerals just by eating food, especially given the fact that today's foods are more devoid of vitamins and nutrients than even a few decades ago. To fulfill your vitamin needs you would have to take in so many calories and carbs that your weight would soar. The best way to get vitamins is to take a high-potency, multivitamin complex.

I don't recommend the commercial brands sold in supermarkets because of the modest amounts of vitamins they contain. Go to a health food store and select a high-potency multivitamin in name brand there. But most importantly, take your vitamins religiously. Many people stop taking their vitamins because pills make them feel nauseous. Few people realize that if you take pills, especially many large-size pills, on an empty stomach, you will probably become nauseated. So don't forget to take your vitamins along with a meal.

When I was an intern, it was common practice for nurses to give pills to patients at 6:00 A.M., well before breakfast. Half an hour later, when I was making my rounds, many of the patients would develop nausea caused by taking pills on an empty stomach. Then I would have to give them yet another pill for nausea. It would have been so much easier to give the pills to the patients after breakfast and avoid nausea altogether.

You will see that my program includes quite a few supplements at quite high dosages. I recommend that you take half to two-thirds of your daily dosages at lunch. The balance should be taken at dinner.

The only exceptions are the fatty acids (fish oil), which should be taken in the morning.

Note: A good multivitamin complex can give you many but not all of the vitamins and other supplements I recommend. Check the label on the multivitamin and look for the recommended supplements. Then fill in what's missing. I highly recommend the vitamins that can be ordered from Life Extension Foundation (800-544-4440). Their vitamins and supplements are of very high quality and priced competitively.

FATTY ACIDS

Let us begin with essential fatty acids, perhaps the most important and certainly the most underrepresented anti-aging supplement in our Western diet.

Essential fatty acid supplementation is profoundly important to fight weight gain, high insulin levels, hunger, tiredness, poor concentration, and yes, even skin aging. Dr. Barry Sears, author of *The Zone,* made a tremendous contribution to the field of nutrition, anti-aging, and wellness when he pointed out the remarkable physiological relevance of long-chain omega-3 fatty acids from fish oil in the production of eicosanoids. Eicosanoids are hormones that are made in each cell of the body. These fragile hormones never enter circulation; in fact, they never even leave the cell, but they exert a controlling influence over all the body's hormonal systems.

There are two basic categories of eicosanoids, and simply put, we can call them "good" E and "bad" E. If the balance of E in your cells is tilted toward the bad E, you are more likely to develop chronic disease. You may age faster, gain weight, and struggle with high insulin and faster-aging skin. On the other hand, if your balance is tilted toward the good E, you have a very good chance for wellness, slower aging processes, weight and insulin control, and better skin.

What determines the ratio of good versus bad E in the cells? It's the ratio of two essential fatty acids in the blood: the ratio of arachidonic acid and eicosapentaenoic acid (AA/EPA).

The only way we can influence the ratio of good E to bad E is to fortify our diet with long-chain omega-3 from fish oil. Unfortunately, there is no other source that can supply long-chain omega-3. Vegetable oils are unable to help here because they are *short-chain* omega-3 molecules. The *long-chain* omega-3 fatty acid can only come from fish. There is no drug that can favorably change the proportion of good E and bad E, and we do not make the ingredients in our system, so we either ingest the right fatty acids or live with the detrimental consequences of chronic E imbalance.

A surprising majority of people live in a chronic state of deficiency of long-chain omega-3. The good news is that according to science, high-dose fish oil will have a greater impact on your state of youth, health, and longevity than any other dietary intervention you can possibly take. A greater control of your insulin levels goes hand in hand with increasing your intake of high-dose fish oils as well, because excess insulin can induce the body to make more omega-6 fatty acids, therefore upsetting the favorable balance of good E and bad E.

Just how much fish oil do you need? A very important question because, as you know, in nutritional supplementation, everything rises and falls on the percentages. You must have at least three grams of long-chain omega-3. One six-ounce serving of salmon is only one gram. To get the dose you need, you would have to have salmon three times a day, and the salmon has to be wild salmon, not farm-raised. Farm-raised salmon may achieve exactly the opposite of what you are looking for. (Most farm-raised salmon has a lot of arachidonic acid, which gives rise to more bad E than to good E.)

The other problem with eating lots of wild salmon is that if you eat large quantities you will ingest dangerously high levels of mercury, DDT, and PCB, which are known carcinogens. Whatever toxins we dump in the ocean eventually end up in the fish.

How can you get adequate levels of long-chain omega-3 without eating salmon all day and ingesting known carcinogens and mercury? The answer is pharmacological-grade fish oil. It is best to have your three grams of fish supplement at the beginning of the day so you can best be prepared to meet the physiological stresses of the day. You can take it in capsule form (eight to twelve capsules a day), but it's easier to take a spoonful of oil and be done with it. The pharmacological-grade fish oil is highly purified, so it contains negligible amounts of mercury, PCB, and DDT, and it should not give you gastrointestinal problems. Dr. Barry Sears sells a very good pure fish oil that I recommend. From a caloric point of view, the three grams of oil you need amount to about forty calories, which is not significant. The benefits of overall health, insulin control, and anti-aging are well worth it.

Including fish oil as part of your daily diet will give you more energy, both physically and mentally. The preponderance of good E will give you better oxygen transfer from blood to brain, to muscle, and to heart. This will translate to increased energy levels, better mental focus, and better circulation.

Your skin quality may improve as well. Skin may be more supple because of improved blood flow, and increased good E can combat the dry, frail, thinning skin caused by bad E. Even the strength of your nails and the condition of your hair may change. In fact, your hair and nails can serve as good visual indicators of the balance between the good E and the bad E. Poor, fragile nails and brittle hair quality can indicate an overpreponderance of bad E and can be predictors of premature aging. You *can* change that with high-dose fish oil.

Good E may lessen your appetite for carbs and decrease your insulin release. With less insulin on board you'll experience less hunger and your blood glucose levels may stabilize. Fish oil is very good for treating a faulty glucose metabolism. Diabetes is nonexistent among Eskimos, who consume on average seven to ten grams of fish oil a day. There is no question that the right fats can be instrumental in starting to burn your own fat. Isn't all this a good enough reason is swallow a spoonful of oil?

CARNOSINE

Another powerful anti-aging supplement that many people are not familiar with as of yet is carnosine. This remarkable substance is one of the most important nutrients you can take for protection against the ravages of aging in the form of glycation and protein carbonylation. While most of us are familiar with the oxidative process and anti-oxidants such as vitamins C, A, and E, alphalipoic acid, and CoQ10, most people have never encountered the concept of protein carbonylation and glycation. Glycation refers to the process where glucose attaches itself to the protein, and carbonylation occurs when a carbonyl molecule attaches itself to the protein molecule. Both of these processes modify the protein, and not in a good way. They contribute to the deterioration of our body's proteins. Protein carbonylation and glycation occur to skin cells as well, and this is one of the main intrinsic reason why the skin ages.

Recent research identifies carnosine as the most promising broad-spectrum shield that is effective against nearly all of the chemical processes that destroy protein and make us age. The only problem is that our level of carnosine rapidly declines as we age. The main dietary source of carnosine is red meat and, of course these days, few people eat a lot of red meat. So we must take carnosine as a supplement.

For carnosine supplementation to be effective, you have to take at least 1,000 mg per day, all at once. If you take less, an enzyme will digest your carnosine supplement as you take it, and it will do you no good. However, if you take more than a 1,000 mg at any one time, the enzyme cannot digest it completely, so you have some left to do work. Carnosine in a multivitamin is present in modest amounts only (50 mg–100 mg), so you will have to take it as a separate supplement. (Check out Life Extension for good quality and prices.)

ANTIOXIDANTS

The oxidative process, the other culprit in aging, is addressed by substances known as antioxidants. Antioxidants can be vitamins, minerals, amino acids, hormones, and enzymes. All these different categories of antioxidants can disarm damaging free radicals to some modest degree and protect protein and DNA, our genetic message system. Unfortunately, only perhaps a third of all antioxidant activity can be influenced by diet and supplements. The rest of your antioxidant protection capacity is inherent in your genes. I recommend that the following antioxidants be taken daily.

Vitamin C
It is nearly impossible to obtain all our vitamin C needs from dietary sources, so it is wise to supplement. Surprisingly, human beings are one of the very few animals (along with guinea pigs and a certain songbird called a red vented bulbul) who do not manufacture vitamin C. A goat, for instance, makes as much as 13,000 mg of vitamin C per day. This makes you wonder how experts could have come up with the paltry 50 mg of the minimum recommended dose for human beings!

Vitamin C is an essential cofactor in collagen production in the skin. That means if vitamin C is lacking, there is little collagen production in the skin. Topical application assures better vitamin C concentration on the skin. However, there has to be a certain blood level of vitamin C as well, to maintain good skin from the inside out. So vitamin C is not something you can skimp on. You must take 2,000 mg a day—divided between lunch and dinner.

Your daily vitamin C intake should occur in conjunction with 500 to 1,000 mg per day of *bioflavonoids.* Bioflavonoids are antioxidant pigments from plants such as pycnogenol, grapeseed extract, quercetin, and rutin. Bioflavonoids enhance the benefits and the absorption of vitamin C, so it's best to take them together. See more on bioflavonoids below.

Bioflavonoids

As I mentioned earlier, bioflavonoids are pigments from plants and fruits that protect us from free-radical damage. There are many different bioflavonoids. Some of the most important ones are: *Pycnogenol* (at 400 mg per day), a powerful free-radical scavenger with known anticancer functions. Pycnogenol keeps collagen elastic, improves vessel walls, and may protect against stroke and dementia. *Quercetin* shows anticancer and cardioprotective properties. *Rutin* can inhibit tumor growth and improve hypercholesterolemia and circulation. *Resveratrol* is one of the key antioxidants. Derived from red grapes, it is thought to be responsible for the "French paradox"—the fact that French people have one of the lowest rates of cardiovascular ailments, while consuming a high-fat diet complemented with daily red wine.

Vitamin E

Vitamin E is another critical element in the antioxidant puzzle. Take at least 400 IU of *alpha tocopherol,* the most common form of Vitamin E. If you can, it's better to take a combination of the more potent *gamma tocopherol* with alpha tocopherol and beta tocotrienols. The ideal combination may be 400 to 600 IU of alpha tocopherol (natural version), with 200 to 300 mg of gamma tocopherol and 100 mg of beta tocotrienols. Read the label and look for a combination of all these different forms of vitamin E.

Scientific evidence about the benefits of vitamin E is so overwhelming that there is just no excuse not to take it. Taking vitamin E supplements daily will significantly reduce your risk of heart disease and stroke. Vitamin E is also a cancer fighter, it mitigates symptoms of arthritis, and so much more.

Vitamin E helps your skin stay youthful by protecting against UV radiation. However, taking vitamin E does not excuse you from using daily sunscreen. Scientific evidence shows that vitamin E may be instrumental in helping you fight aging at a cellular level. Long before we see outward evidence of aging such as wrinkles, gray hair, etc., the damage begins at a cellular level. The accumulation of age pigment called lipo-fuscin in skin cells (dark spots), brain cells, and the heart is a direct result of lipid peroxidation. Vitamin E can slow this process significantly.

CoQ10

The recommended dose of this antioxidant is 100 mg per day with meals. CoQ10 is present in literally all cells and is actually also known as ubiquinone, derived from the word ubiquitous.

About 95 percent of all cellular energy (along with your perceived energy level) comes from structures in the cells called mitochondria. Mitchondria are cellular powerhouses that convert sugars and fats into energy via the oxidative process. CoQ10 deactivates some of the free radicals that are released during the energy-generating process. At the same time, it takes part in the energy-gaining process. We do produce CoQ10 for ourselves; however, the problem is that the production of CoQ10 declines by about 50 percent by middle age, and—you guessed right—so does our energy level. That is why it is critical for people over age thirty-five to take CoQ10.

Acetyl-l-Carnitine (ALC)

I strongly recommend this naturally occurring amino acid at 2,000 mg per day. Research shows that acetyl-l-carnitine helps with memory; it slows and even, to some extent, reverses short-term memory loss and neurological damage from stroke and depression. It is not an antioxidant per se, but its anti-aging qualities put ALC into this category.

Alpha Lipoic Acid

I recommend 100 to 200 mg per day. Make sure to take it with a significant amount of food because it is both fat and water soluble and because it can be very irritating on an empty stomach. Alpha lipoic acid is one of the key antioxidants to supplement because this is our only way to boost the level of glutathion—nature's master antioxidant.

Glutathion has been shown to be essential to slowing down cellular aging.

Beta-carotene

The daily recommended dose is 25,000 IU. Beta-carotene is the substance from which the body makes vitamin A. Beta-carotene and the mixed carotenoids are powerful antioxidants and are intimately involved in the aging process. It is best to take them together. Fortunately, they are found together in most good multivitamins. Beta-carotene supplementation can decrease your chances of a heart attack by as much as 40 percent.

B VITAMINS AND FOLIC ACID

It is difficult to obtain adequate quantities of B vitamins from your diet, so it is best to take them in a multivitamin complex. As we age, our stomach secretes less and less hydrochloric acid. This reduced secretion has a profound influence on our body's ability to absorb some of the B vitamins, especially vitamin B_{12} and folic acid. So B complex supplementation in older adults is no longer an option, it is a necessity. I recommend the following dosages of vitamin B and folic acid.

Folic acid—800 mcg

Niacin (vitamin B_3)—100 mg

Pantothenic acid—2,000 mcg

Riboflavin (vitamin B_2)—50 mg

Thiamine (vitamin B_1)—50 mg

Vitamin B_6—50 mg

Vitamin B_{12}—600 mcg

MINERAL SUPPLEMENTS

Calcium plays a key role in preventing osteoporosis; however, the vast majority of the adult population takes less than the necessary dose of calcium, which is 1,500 to 1,800 mg, depending on age and sex. One of the best forms of calcium is calcium citrate. Then again, calcium may do very little in the absence of other minerals and vitamins such as *vitamin D₃, magnesium, manganese,* and *zinc,* so it is best to take them in the same formulation. A formulation marketed by the Life Extension Foundation contains all the necessary ingredients for proper calcium supplementation. Unfortunately, even adequate amounts of calcium will not protect you from osteoporosis in the absence of estrogen. Menopausal women should see their doctors and have a bone scan regularly to make sure they have adequate amounts of calcium in the bones.

Chromium is a critically important element in insulin metabolism. The minimum daily dose is 200 mg. It is generally found in multivitamins. If not, take it separately to help control insulin.

Magnesium is an essential component of bone formation. It is involved in lowering blood pressure, and it has a calming effect on the nervous system. Stress conditions use up more magnesium than normal. Chocolate cravings may be a sign of magnesium deficiency because chocolate is a good source of magnesium. The recommended daily dose of magnesium is 1,200 mg.

Manganese is an important antioxidant and trace mineral. It acts as an activator of many enzymes and is indispensable. Manganese is involved in cholesterol metabolism and improves the functioning of the immune system. The recommended dose of manganese is 100 mg per day.

Selenium is an essential trace mineral and an antioxidant that works synergistically with vitamin E. The recommended daily dose in 200 mcg.

Zinc is one of the central minerals involved in countless physiological functions. Many things can go wrong if you are zinc-deficient, from faulty protein synthesis to problems with eicosonoid synthesis, so please take at least 50 mg of chelated zinc a day.

In general, it is best to take take your minerals in a chelated form for superior absorption.

HYALURONIC ACID

This acid plays a vital role in maintaining and regulating moisture in our cells, helping to transport nutrients into the cells and, just as importantly, remove metabolic waste. Getting rid of these harmful toxins also helps eliminate the buildup of lipofuscin pigment, which causes age spots. The daily recommended dose is 10 mg.

DR. DENESE'S ANTI-AGING DIET AND SUPPLEMENT PLAN AT A GLANCE

MORNING:

· Protein-only breakfast. NO CARBS except some low–Glycemic Index berries or fruits if you don't need to lose any weight.

· Three grams of fish oil in any way that makes it palatable for you.

· Fiber.

MIDAFTERNOON:

· Protein: chicken, fish, turkey. Low–Glycemic Index vegetables, green salads. No carbs if possible.

· Half daily dose of supplements, to include carnosine, vitamin C, vitamin E, CoQ10, acetyl-l-carnitine, alphalipoic acid, vitamin B, vitamin B_{12}, folic acid, beta-carotene, calcium, chromium, magnesium, manganese, and zinc in a high-potency-vitamin supplement.

LATE-AFTERNOON SNACK:

· Low–Glycemic Index fruits and some other foods from the low–Glycemic Index chart.

EVENING:

· Protein, low–Glycemic Index vegetables, green salads, minimal carbs, and low–Glycemic Index fruits.

· No potatoes, rice, breads, or sweets at any point.

· The balance of daily dose of supplements.

NO CARBOHYDRATES FOR THREE HOURS BEFORE SLEEP.

CHAPTER FOUR

THE DENESE SIX-STEP PROGRAM FOR AGELESS SKIN

Now that you are starting to combat the aging process from the inside, you can begin working on the outside—the skin. Your face is the first thing people notice when they look at you, and it unfortunately shows the telltale signs of aging the quickest. But now you can help your face look younger, longer. Just following my easy six-step program will make some changes in the condition of your skin.

The world of beauty has always been filled with fantastic claims and promises. I am not going to insult your intelligence by promising that if you follow my six-step plan you will have an equivalent of a face-lift. You have heard that before and, in spite of your best efforts, it did not happen. I won't make that promise because a face-lift is impossible to deliver by topical means.

However, I can promise:

- a visible change in the look of lines and wrinkles

- a significant visual improvement in pore size

- a more supple, youthful, dewy skin tone and a complexion that feels less dry

- a dramatic improvement in the appearance of dry lines around the eyes and mouth

- a remarkable visual change in the evenness of color and the return of a youthful, glowing radiance that you thought was lost forever

And I promise that if you follow these steps as described, you will see results in weeks.

FACE THE FACTS: LOOK IN THE MIRROR

The good news is that there are only a handful of changes that happen to our skin as we age—eight, to be exact, not counting any of the medical skin conditions that are beyond the scope of this book. So we have eight age-related skin problems to solve:

1. lines and wrinkles

2. enlarged pores

3. clogged pores and bumpiness under the skin

4. skin turning sallow, dull, lacking radiance

5. dark discolorations such as age spots; sun spots; or large, amorphous, dark discolorations (melasma) and dark spots on former acne sites

6. red capillaries or generalized redness around the nose and cheeks

7. sagging around the jawline and under the chin

8. thinning, dry skin

Based on recent scientific advances, your topical skin care may be able to do far more than you think to undo the appearance of skin damage and prevent age-related changes. The Denese Six-Step Program can deal with the majority of them very successfully. However, the only way you and I will succeed is if you are willing to give up most of the traditional skin-care ideas that the cosmetics establishment has fed you. You may not have a lot to lose, since traditional skin care gives you traditional results, which, traditionally, are minimal.

To begin, however, you have to part with the conventional idea of **cream-based** skin care altogether and realize that the magic jar of cream that can address all of your skin-care concerns is nothing but a scientific fallacy.

You have to give up the idea that skin care is a simple two-step process: clean, and put on the magic overnight cream.

You may also have to realize that skin care does not *always* have to feel good.

Last but not least, you have to accept the fact that wearing sun protection every day of the year is essential—rain or shine.

However, if you do accept these simple ideas, the Denese Six-Step Program is the only skin-care program you will ever need.

THE DENESE SIX-STEP PROGRAM

Based on state-of-the-art medical knowledge, I have identified six phases of skin care—phases you will need to complete every night, in precise order, no skipping, to successfully address the eight visual signs of aging skin.

1. *The cleansing phase.*

2. *The exfoliating phase.*

3. *The skin-stimulating phase* encourages the skin's own collagen-building machinery and repair mechanism to soften the look of lines and wrinkles. This is ideally done with a thin water-consistency serum, rich in ingredients that easily permeate the skin. This step does not feel particularly moisturizing and it may leave your skin feeling dry and tingly.

4. *The skin-building phase* moisturizes via lipid (fat) soluble vitamins, nutrients, antioxidants, retinal, and essential fatty acids.

5. *The skin-sealing phase* moisturizes and prevents water loss by sealing the skin. It feels good and soothing and helps repair the skin lipid barrier.

6. *The skin-protection phase* consists of using SPF 30 sun protection daily in the morning and throughout the day, rain or shine, every day of the year.

If you only do the skin sealing step your skin will feel good on the way but you may not get very far in terms of results. If you only do the skin building step you will achieve results, but your skin may feel dry and show more dry lines temporarily.

If you build the skin first, then seal it, you will have the best of both worlds.

PHASE 1: THE CLEANSING PHASE

Look inside your medicine cabinet. Do you have a cleanser and a toner and, more importantly, do you use *both* every day? I have patients who tell me that they wash their face with soap and water every day. This works for the twenty-year-old girl on a soap commercial, but believe me, the last time she probably washed her face with soap and water was during the filming of the TV ad. This may have worked for *you* in your twenties, but if you are older than twenty-five, I absolutely do not recommend soap. The pH of soap is not what your skin needs; it will dry out your skin without cleaning it properly.

You need a lot more science in your cleansing phase.

A good cleanser has a pH close to that of skin. It does not dry your skin, and it has some AHA (alpha-hydroxy acids) or BHA (beta-hydroxy acids) content. The reason for AHA/BHA is that these chemicals open pores, exfoliate, dissolve oily plugs, and take off some of the old, dry skin cells from the surface. A good AHA/BHA cleanser will do that without stripping your skin and leaving it feeling tight and dry.

Here's a tip: There's no need to spend a great deal of money on cleanser. Don't fall for a list of fancy ingredients. Why? In the first place, you wash a cleanser off, so you will not enjoy the benefits of the ingredients for very long. Second, in most products made by the major cosmetics companies, the good and sexy ingredients (for example, vitamin C, vitamin A, CoQ10, etc.) are there in tiny quantities. The reason is simple: economics. Cleansers are sold in large bottles (six to eight ounces, typically). The ingredients are very costly, so most of the major cosmetics houses put minimal amounts of the active ingredients in the mix. Don't buy a fancy, expensive cleanser. Just find one you like. The right cleanser should leave your skin feeling soft and refreshed, not dry, pulled, or tight in any way.

Another tip: despite what the cosmetics ads tell you, water-free, leave-on cleansers (the milky cleansers that you apply with a cotton ball and don't wash off) are *not* good for your skin. Unless you are elderly, with paper-thin, fragile, dry skin, this is not for you. It may lead to clogged pores, blackheads, and a skin that lacks any radiant glow.

Other than that, most cleansers will be fine, because your cleanser is just the beginning of your cleaning process.

Toners are the second step in the cleansing process. Why do you need a toner? A reasonable question. I asked it myself before I went to medical school and started my medical practice. What good can it possibly do?

Try this test: Go to your medicine cabinet, take out a cleanser, and wash off your makeup. Wash as you normally would when you are sleepy at night. Do not cheat. Now take a cotton ball or wipe, soak it in toner, and rub your face with it. Look at the wipe. If you see makeup residue, dirt, and grime, you are seeing one good reason to use toner.

A toner provides the second step of cleansing: it removes the dirt that the cleanser missed. In fact, it is better to cleanse in two steps than one. If you expect to take everything off with the cleanser, you are asking too much from the cleanser. Also, the mechanical rubbing with the toner-soaked cotton ball takes off more dirt than no rubbing at all.

Do not fall for expensive toners that make outrageous claims. Remember, a very small amount of the key ingredients that the toner boasts about on the label are in a large bottle of toner. I am not suggesting that all cleansers and toners are the same, or that you should buy the least expensive toner. However, if you have to economize on your skin-care regimen, this is where it will hurt the least.

But remember, after cleansing and toning you are still not finished with cleaning your face. The most important part is still to come.

PHASE 2: THE EXFOLIATING PHASE

It is almost impossible to exfoliate too much provided you follow the directions on a product label and use some common sense. But how do you know if you are exfoliating enough? Look in the mirror. If you have clogged pores around the nose or forehead, bumpiness under the skin, if your face lacks radiance, looks dull and sallow, or if you see dry lines and enlarged pores, then you are **not** exfoliating enough. All these problems can be successfully addressed by proper exfoliation. The vast majority of adults underexfoliate.

Don't buy into the myth that an AHA/BHA cleanser and toner is all the exfoliation you need. Based on my clinical experience as a doctor, this is *completely untrue.* This dangerous lie may lead to skin that is dull, sallow, has clogged pores, and lacks radiance.

If you think that all you have to do is buy a face wash with glycolic acid that promises exfoliation and now you are exfoliating enough, have met all the needs of your skin, think again. Typically a glycolic face wash (AHA/BHA) contains 1 percent glycolic acid. You may need to use ten times that strength daily.

I can understand how you may be misguided about this very important practice. But by the time you finish reading this book, you will be an expert on the subject.

Have you ever heard that exfoliation or "overexfoliation" may thin the skin in the long run?

It seems to make sense, right? It seems intuitive to think that if you remove layers of skin, the skin will grow thin. However, one of the most important and basic ideas you learn if you study the skin at the scientific level is that the skin is a dynamic organ, and *the more you wear it down the more it grows.* Any skin-care professional who tells you otherwise is truly *not* qualified to take care of your skin. In fact, you can use this question as a test to gauge the experience and expertise of a skin-care professional.

Exfoliation is truly the key building block toward your goal of flawless skin for three reasons:

1. Exfoliation may stimulate cellular turnover, may encourage the skin's own collagen building, and may improve skin thickness. Skin thickness is what ultimately improves the look of lines and wrinkles; thicker skin is less wrinkled.

2. If you have a thick layer of *dead* cells on top of your skin, how will the precious collagen-building nutrients in your skin-care products reach your skin? Exfoliation creates the ability to transport the key ingredients of skin-care products to their destination.

3. Exfoliation is your final cleansing phase. It is your last chance to open up clogged pores before they become little bumps under your skin.

When we are young our skin exfoliates rapidly. Dead skin cells are naturally and steadily sloughed off. As we grow older, the natural exfoliation process becomes more and more sluggish. Without extra exfoliation, the skin turns ashen, dull, and sallow. It loses the fabulous translucent, radiant look of youth because there is an accumulation of dead skin cells on the surface of the skin.

I have heard people say that they don't exfoliate because their skin is too dry. One of the common reasons why people suffer from dry skin is that they have a thick layer of dead skin cells covering the skin surface, so a moisturizer cannot penetrate properly. So if you feel dry, you may need to do exactly what for so long you have believed you should not: exfoliate.

Interestingly enough, my younger patients, in their twenties and thirties, have no trouble with this concept. They exfoliate aggressively, use the serums of the skin-stimulating phase, followed by the sealing creams, and they get excellent results. On the other hand, my middle-aged patients, who most need to understand this medical concept, are more resistant to the idea. I understand that it is not easy to shed the long-held traditional view about feel-good, low-yield skin care, even if it does not deliver what it promises. I understand how counterintuitive it may be to use strong glycolic acid pads and strong serums on your face every night if you have frail, thin skin and are accustomed to rich creams that do nothing but smell good. However, try to keep an open mind. Few people realize that skin is often dry because of a thick layer of dry, dead skin cells that must be removed before moisture can penetrate into the face.

LIVING PROOF

When sixty-four-year-old Rose first came to my office, she had dry, sallow-looking skin that was crying for moisture. The lines around her eyes and on her cheeks stood out sharply every time she smiled.

"No matter what cream I use or how much of it I apply, my skin still feels dry," she told me.

For many years, Rose had been washing her face twice a day with a soap that she believed was gentle and moisturizing. She'd never considered using a cleanser that contained a glycolic acid ingredient. She knew glycolic acid was an exfoliant, and she was convinced that any wearing down of her skin would only exacerbate her problem and create even more dryness and irritation. She was shocked when I suggested that she begin using glycolic pads.

"One of the most common contributing factors of dry skin is a thick layer of old, dry, dead cells that are sitting on top of your face, blocking the penetration of moisture," I told her. "You wouldn't take a shower with a raincoat on, but that is what you do when you try to moisturize without removing the old cells." I explained that exfoliating with the pads once a day would revitalize her skin and prepare it to absorb all the benefits of good water-based and lipid-based skin-building serums. Then, as a last step in her regimen, I instructed her to apply a rich cream to seal in moisture.

Rose was skeptical, but she reluctantly agreed to give the new regimen a try.

"If extreme redness and irritation develop, you can scale back and take a few days' break," I said. "But keep in mind that even if redness and irritation occur, these will by no means hurt your skin. This reaction will resolve itself in a short time, and your skin will begin to look much better."

Three weeks later, Rose returned to my office with a new glow about her. Her skin was significantly softer, and the lines around the eyes and cheeks no longer had sharp edges to them.

"The dryness went away," she said with a very happy smile. "My skin looks much less lined now. I feel like I took ten years off my face."

How do you exfoliate properly?

Let me put it this way: If you had an esthetician for a roommate and she gave you an AHA or BHA peel every third day or a microdermabrasion scrub every week, that might be enough exfoliation, but still not too much. So what do you do if you live with your husband and he is not interested in giving you daily skin peels? The best thing is to try to seek out a home version of a doctor's glycolic acid exfoliating treatment that you can use regularly, per the enclosed instructions. One of the most effective ways I have found to exfoliate is with an **8 percent to 10 percent glycolic acid pad** every night. This does not require a prescription, although it is not easy to find. You might have an easier time getting them at doctors' offices. The acidity level of the product is very significant in terms of product effectiveness. My exfoliating pads, Facial Firming Pads by Dr. Denese, are very popular. Dr. Perricone's Pore Refining Toner Pads and DDF Glycolic 10% Daily Cleansing Pads are also very good. When I came out with my glycolic pads, there were no others on the market. They are now becoming very popular, and I'm happy to see this efficient exfoliation device growing more widely available.

Please, do not fall for the inexpensive variety of facial pads that are readily obtainable at commercial drugstores. These pads usually contain a fraction of the glycolic strength that you need. They are widely advertised and easy to find but are not for you. The label may promise all the right results you are hoping for in a skin-care product, but chances are you may never get the results because the product may not be strong enough.

Unfortunately, companies are not obligated to list on the label the percentage of glycolic acid in the product. Even if they list the glycolic percentage, the acidity level (or pH) is also a decisive factor, and that is not listed on the jar. So how can you tell if the glycolic pad is strong enough for you? It's easy to tell. Just test it on your face. The right strength of glycolic pad will have a slight sting. That is how you know it's working. No sting, no result. Your skin will soon get used to the acid, and the sting will go away in a few weeks. That's supposed to happen. You do not have to look for a stronger product. But if the pad never tingles your skin, even at the beginning, it is not the right product for you.

Remember, you are the best judge to know if something works or not. Do not read the promises on the box; read your face in the mirror in a few weeks. That is all you need to know.

A weak glycolic peel is just another skin-care conspiracy lie. You think you are doing the right thing for your skin, and you achieve nothing or very little. The right daily glycolic acid peel pad is such a powerful tool that you should see a result from it in about two to three weeks. If you see no positive changes in that time, the glycolic acid peel pad you are using is not strong enough. Look for these changes:

- improvement in the look of pores and lines

- clearer skin with fewer bumps

- improvement in radiance and glow

You may ask: Don't skin-care companies know that the exfoliants they sell are too weak? Don't the cosmetics companies know what strength to use? Of course they do, but once again, it's a matter of economics. Many people, if they feel the slightest sting from a pad, bring it back. Some even try to sue. They do not realize that they *should* feel a slight sting. As far as cosmetics companies are concerned, it is cheaper to disappoint you than to handle returns and deal with legal matters.

A note on salicylic acid-based acne pads. By law, salicylic acid (BHA) can only be sold at 2 percent strength without a prescription, which, on its own, is not sufficient for adequate exfoliation. Look for one that is fortified with glycolic acid as well.

There are also glycolic acid–based exfoliating creams on the market designed to be left on overnight. Many of them are weak, and I do not like the principle of exfoliating and then leaving the debris on the skin. I think it is better to exfoliate and then wipe off dead skin cells and makeup residue with a pad and throw it away. Also, this way you have created a clean surface to absorb the other important ingredients you put on your skin at night.

Once or twice a week, I recommend using a microdermabrasion cream in addition to the pads. Look for microdermabrasion creams with very fine granules. Estée Lauder So Polished Exfoliating Scrub is an excellent product. Also try Botanical Microdermabrasion Cream,

SEEING IS BELIEVING

When you have purchased the right glycolic pad, one that tingles a bit when you use it, try this experiment.

Wash your face and use a toner as you would normally. Then take a pad and wipe one side of your face with it. Then take another pad, rinse it out, removing all the glycolic solution on it, so it is saturated in just water, and wipe the other side of your face. Which of the pads has come off with more dirt? I have shown this experiment to hundreds of patients, and the glycolic pad is always significantly dirtier than the one rinsed in water.

Which would you rather use?

Dr. Brandt Exfoliation in a Jar, L'Oréal Refinish Microdermabrasion Kit, and my own Doctor's Microdermabrasion Cream. Avoid any dermabrasion product that contains coarse particles, such as apricot shell, that can scratch the skin. The object is to *micropolish* the skin without scratching or irritating it.

There are many handheld, battery-operated machines on the market called microdermabrasion machines. Save your money. You do not need any such device. The machines do nothing that you can't accomplish with your hands. In fact, your hands can do a far better job, reaching into every nook and cranny around the nose—the machines often miss these areas entirely. It's my understanding at this time that the FDA is even considering forbidding the use of the name "microdermabrasion" on these gadgets, since the name may mislead the public into believing that the machines offer the same treatment as professional microdermabrasion. This, of course, is most certainly *not* true.

PHASE 3: THE SKIN-STIMULATING PHASE

Now you are ready to stimulate the skin. In this phase, by applying a serum that feeds the skin water-soluble ingredients, you will address the appearance of the lines and wrinkles, enlarged pores, and loss of firmness and elasticity that occur with aging. The common denominator of all these problems is a gradual loss of collagen and collagen breakdown. Collagen is the major skin protein, responsible for elasticity. The ultimate goal in skin care is to encourage the skin's own collagen-producing machinery and stimulate collagen repair. Essentially, all scientific active ingredients are aiming in the direction of collagen buildup.

In my opinion, the best form to supply the important ingredients to the skin, to assure better delivery is a serum.

I have made this point earlier, and I'll be reiterating it throughout this book, because this is the take-home message that is so important.

The skin-care establishment has led you to believe that a magic cream exists that will solve it all. It will stimulate the skin to make more collagen, fill in the wrinkles, and smooth and comfort at the same time. But a cream that can do it all, even in theory, is a *scientific impossibility.* A cream can *either* build the skin to fill in lines, but leave you a bit dry, *or* it can seal and moisturize the skin and make you feel good. *It cannot fulfill both functions at the same time.*

The reason is simple: If a cream is a good moisturizer, the very particles that make the cream a good moisturizer will, to a large extent, block the way of absorption of those ingredients that are intended to stimulate the skin's own collagen-making machinery, perform antioxidant functions, and exfoliate. If the cream lacks moisturizing capacity, it may allow the penetration of these key ingredients, which is a great positive; however, this cream will feel dry, irritating, and miserable, which is a huge negative.

The bottom line is that a cream can either feel good, but do precious little, or feel uncomfortable, but do everything modern science has to offer.

So do we have to choose between feeling good and looking good?

Hardly. Although the skin-stimulating and skin-building phases by themselves may leave your skin somewhat irritated, especially initially, the skin-sealing phase feels good. So if you stimulate and build first, then seal, you will have the best of both worlds.

The skin-care industry has not paid much attention to creating a high-powered, highly penetrating, thin, water-based serum because such a product may not have much curb appeal. People expect a skin product to feel moisturizing, so a serum that doesn't feel moisturizing is not automatically a good seller. You may have difficulty locating one. Doctors' offices are one place to go. I make products called Cellular Firming Serum, Growth Factor Serum, and a 15 percent vitamin C serum. You can also look in your health food store or check online. I like Skinceuticals Serum 15 a lot, as well as Cellex C High Potency Serum.

A serum is water-based if one of the first ingredients is water and it has a thin consistency. Other ingredients to look for include carnosine, resveratrol, bioactive oligopeptides, copper, vitamin C, and vitamin B complex.

I especially like carnosine and strongly recommend it. Several studies have found that it has a remarkable revitalizing and regenerating effect on skin fibroblasts. And believe me, skin fibroblasts are your friends. They make fresh collagen and elastin in the skin. Carnosine is a dipeptide, a very small entity containing amino acids. This translates into easy access into the skin. Carnosine research is very new, so you may not find this ingredient in many skin-care products. Presented in a thin, water-based serum, carnosine is extremely beneficial in an arsenal of anti-aging weapons.

Resveratrol, a substance extracted from grapes and plants, is another ingredient that, recent scientific studies have shown, may hold some remarkable benefits for skin cells.

To the best of my knowledge, there is only one serum on the market that contains carnosine, in addition to a full range of antioxidants, and that is my patent-pending product called Age Control Serum.

PHASE 4: THE SKIN-BUILDING PHASE

This phase of your skin-care regimen requires a serum that is lipid-based. This serum is used *in addition* to the water-based serum because it provides a way to deliver other important collagen-building ingredients that are soluble only in lipids (fats). You can easily identify a lipid-based serum by looking at the ingredients list—it will not contain water (at least not as one of the prominent ingredients, although it may appear near the end of the ingredients list). Lipid-based serums are thicker and more moisturizing. Look for ones that contain important ingredients such as retinol, vitamin E, essential fatty acids, linoleic acid, Omega 3, and ceramides, which are lipids very similar to the skin's own lipids.

This lipid-based serum performs the very important function in your skin care of re-creating the all-important skin lipid barrier, which serves the vital function of keeping water in the skin. The lipid barrier is a layer of fat molecules that line up right under the surface of the skin in the stratum corneum and form a tight chain, much like a picket fence, in two rows, facing each other. Unfortunately, as we grow older, the skin lipid barrier breaks down (it also can break down from harsh soaps), so the picket fence is not so perfect anymore. The skin becomes increasingly dry.

To re-create the skin lipid barrier, it is best to use the identical lipid molecules that nature intended, which is exactly what is provided in advanced ceramides, essential fatty acids, and linoleic and linolinic acids. If you use anything other than the identical skin lipids (e.g., mineral oils, plant lipids, or lanolin), you may not be able to mend the picket fence properly because the strange lipid molecules will not fit properly in the chain. In fact, the ill-fitting molecules may even clog the skin.

Elizabeth Arden has a ceramide serum that is good. It's called Bye-Lines Anti-Aging Serum. My own Hydro Shield Ultra Moisturizing Serum is rich in ceramide and essential fatty acids, such as Omega 3, so it feels deliciously moisturizing.

PHASE 5: THE SKIN-SEALING PHASE

The final touch to seal it all in is the cream. It also has the important function of repairing the protective skin lipid barrier, so that the skin does not lose too much fluid and feel dry, irritated, and show more lines. At this point in your skin-care program, any cream that feels good to you and is not too heavy for your skin is fine. There are many products from which you can choose, in all price ranges. It is best to use a cream that contains skin-identical lipids (ceramides), since they fit into the skin far better than any other plant, animal, or mineral oils, which, as I've explained earlier, may clog the pores. But the most significant treatment benefits of my program come from the skin-stimulating and -building serums; the primary purpose of the cream is to seal. The most important function of the cream is that it should feel good and make your skin feel soft and moisturized. This is the pampering phase of your skin-care routine.

Everyone's skin is so different in how much sealing effect it needs. Find the cream that is satisfying for your skin and doesn't look shiny for hours. If it remains shiny it means there are oils that are not permeating the skin, and sooner or later it will clog pores and lead to future problems.

In my experience, many younger women overuse creams and choose night creams that are too heavy for their skin.

How can you tell if a cream is too heavy for you? Again, you need to rely on your own experience. If you find that within three to four weeks of using a cream you see more clogged pores and bumpiness under the skin, the cream is too heavy for you. Stop using it, get a professional exfoliation at a doctor's office (a series of microdermabrasions or chemical peels), and never go back to that cream again.

PHASE 6: THE SKIN-PROTECTION PHASE

Welcome to the new way of life: *SPF 30, 365 days a year.*

I recommend to my patients SPF 30 protection every day, no matter if they are indoors or outdoors and no matter what the season. Finding that degree of sun protection in products may not always be easy, but you should never use less than SPF 15 protection, under any circumstances. It is best to use a day cream with a built-in SPF 30 protection instead of a day cream plus a sunscreen. The reason is that if you have two separate steps, a cream plus a sunscreen, they will dilute each other on the surface of the skin, and the SPF protection level becomes less. It may become as little as the average of the two (0 and 30 = 15). For instance: If you put on a cream in the morning with SPF 0, and then you put on a foundation with SPF 8, you may only have SPF 4 protection on your face. Serums do not need to be calculated into this equation because they absorb into the skin.

YOUR MORNING ROUTINE

My program is designed to be a nighttime routine. It's the best time, so that all the ingredients can work effectively while you are resting. So, you may ask, what should you do in the morning?

The answer is: very little. There's no need to spend more than a few minutes on skin care when you wake. Your first step should be to soak a cotton ball in toner and rub it over your face.

The most important goals that your skin care must achieve during the day are to prevent moisture from evaporating from your skin and to protect your skin from sun exposure. Dry heat, air conditioning, and dry climates all steal moisture from your skin. Your lipid-based serum will do a fine job of putting moisture into your skin. Apply it as your base, then seal it with a good tinted day cream (which should contain many of the same ingredients as a good night cream). I like a cream with a bit of color, so it blends with my skin. Choose one that feels good to you. The right day cream should contain sunscreen protection, be oil-free, light, matte, and blend with your skin color to perfection so you have no excuse not to wear it 365 days a year. Be sure it has SPF 15 protection, at the least, although I think SPF 30 is ideal.

I'm a fan of zinc oxide as a sunscreen because it provides the broadest-spectrum sun protection. Zinc oxide is one of the most superior broad-spectrum sunscreens that address both UVB/UVA rays. The only problem with zinc oxide is that it is hideous pale white. It makes you look like a ghost when you apply it. I've addressed this problem in my sunscreen product by adding melanin, the natural pigment of the skin. The melanin in the cream blends to perfection with any skin color, including all ethnic skins.

So that's it. Six steps that can be completed in less than five minutes at night and two minutes in the morning. I promise that if you follow this regimen, you will see results. Isn't it time to let science work for your skin?

Of course it is.

WHAT TO LOOK FOR

CLEANSER: The best ingredients to seek out in this product are alpha- and beta-hydroxy acids, which are excellent cleaning agents, and other beneficial additions, such as vitamins C and E. However, the key isn't just the ingredients—you rinse them off very quickly—but finding a good cleanser that doesn't leave your skin feeling tight and dry. You should judge your cleanser based on the condition of your skin after you've washed, rinsed, and dried. Your face should feel fresh, clean, and comfortable, not dry or pulled.

TONER: The same criteria apply. An effective toner will have a gentle astringency, yet it should leave your face feeling soft and refreshed. If your skin doesn't feel pulled and dry after you've applied it, it's the right product for you.

EXFOLIANT: The best test, once again, is how it feels on your skin. In this case, it should tingle, at least at first. Look for glycolic acid peel pads with an 8 percent to 10 percent strength solution. Clinical studies of glycolic preparations have shown significant collagen-stimulating and skin-thickness-building action at the right glycolic concentration at the right pH levels. If, the first few times you use it, it just feels like water on a pad and it doesn't have any "bite," you may know that it is *not* strong enough for you. In addition to its skin-building capacity, the pad will exfoliate. If you have dry skin, aggressive exfoliation can remove old skin cells so moisture can reach your skin.

MICRODERMABRASION CREAM: You need this product for additional exfoliation once a week, or twice, if your skin has the tolerance for it. A good microdermabrasion cream should have a rich texture and contain abrasive particles—aluminum oxide or pumice is ideal—but the particles should be very small. Avoid products that contain large grains of any rough or sharp particles. The purpose of this step is to micropolish your face, not scratch it. And the cream should feel good. When you rinse it off, your face should *not* feel tight or dry, but rather smooth, soft, and soothed.

SKIN-STIMULATING SERUM: With this step, use a water-based serum. Water should be listed as the first ingredient. Then look for peptides (which may appear as amino acid or bioactive oligopeptides), carnosine vitamin C (which may appear as L-ascorbic acid), alphalipoic acid, CoQ10, vitamin B_5 complex, hyaluronic acid, grapeseed extract, to name a few of my favorites. If there is some glycolic acid in the formula, it will enhance the effectiveness by helping the serum to penetrate.

SKIN-BUILDING SERUM: At this point you need a lipid-based serum to moisturize and build the skin lipid barrier. Water should *not* be listed at the top of the ingredients list. Look for ceramides (lipids that are identical to your skin lipids), EFAs (essential fatty acids such as linoleic acid), Omega 3, vitamin A (which may appear as retinol), and vitamin E (which may appear as tocotrienol).

With this regimen you are layering your face with all the rich ingredients that are so effective in fighting the signs of aging. You will also want to use skin relaxants for your eye and forehead area. Look for serums or creams that contain the crease relaxer ingredient, argireline.

These serums are scientifically advanced products, and they aren't going to be easily found at the drugstore or health food store. They've become fashionable, but the ingredients are expensive. You can expect to pay a lot for them, but you should also expect to see results. If you don't get them, return the product. On the other hand, don't fall for very-high-priced products in the prestige market. Make sure you're getting the right ingredients. Look for doctors' private label products, check out the most progressive skin-care manufacturers, or browse online. The right products for you are out there.

CREAM: This final application of cream is to seal the skin and rebuild the lipid barrier. First and foremost, a cream should feel good. It should *not* leave your skin feeling dry and your skin should *not* remain shiny for hours after you've applied it. Look for the right level of lipids in the cream that is satisfying to your skin. You can choose from any or all of the rich ingredients above, in the water-based and lipid-based serums, but at this phase of your routine, the penetration will be much less. Ceramides, EFAs, retinol, vitamins C and E, and hyaluronic acid are all excellent ingredients for this last step in your skin-care program.

SUNSCREEN: No matter what time of year, regardless if you are indoors or outdoors, apply sunscreen with an SPF of at least 15— although I prefer SPF 30.

SKIN-CARE FALLACIES

It's not easy to shed the long-held traditional view about feel-good, low-yield skin care, even if it does not deliver what it promises. I understand how counterintuitive it may be to use strong glycolic acid pads and strong serums on your face every night if you have frail, thin skin and you are accustomed to rich creams that do little else but smell good.

The cosmetics establishment would like every woman to continue to believe the following statements:

- An AHA/BHA cleanser and toner are all the exfoliation you need.

- Skin care is a simple two-step process: clean and put on the magic cream.

- One cream is all you need to build the skin and moisturize it at the same time.

- Microdermabrasion creams offer the same treatment as professional microdermabrasion machines.

None of these statements is true. When you, at last, give up believing in these falsehoods, you can begin to really meet all of your skin-care needs and enjoy an agelessly beautiful complexion for life.

CHAPTER FIVE

WINNING THE WRINKLE WAR

Now let us look in the mirror and inspect our skin. Remember, the good news is that there are only a handful of things that happen to our skin as we age—eight, to be exact, not counting any of the medical skin conditions that are beyond the scope of our discussion. I'll repeat them here:

1. lines and wrinkles

2. enlarged pores

3. clogged pores and bumpiness under the skin

4. skin turning sallow, dull, lacking radiance

5. dark discolorations such as age spots; sun spots; dark spots on former acne sites; or large, amorphous dark discolorations (melasma)

6. red capillaries or generalized redness around the nose and cheeks

7. sagging around the jawline and under the chin

8. thinning, dry skin

For most of us, the most alarming of these signs—the one that makes us *feel* old—is the sudden appearance of lines and wrinkles.

My six-step program shows you how to improve and preserve the suppleness of your skin to reduce fine lines, blemishes, enlarged pores, and uneven tones. But to eliminate wrinkles, the deeper effects of aging that have already begun to take their toll, you may have to go farther.

THE ANATOMY OF A WRINKLE

A wrinkle is made up of three parts:

- the skin component

- the underlying muscle component

- the subcutaneous fat and connective tissue components

This information is important for you to know for far more than mere academic interest. It's critical to your understanding of how wrinkles can be treated in the right ways. It's also critical to protect you from falling for deceptive advertising and being taken in by before-and-after pictures that demonstrate skin-care products. *Believe me, cosmetics companies definitely do not want you to realize what I am about to tell you.*

Look in the mirror. Keep your face straight, don't smile, and focus on the area around your eyes. Do you see any wrinkles? You probably don't see many—perhaps none at all. Now, smile broadly, hold it, and look again. Your reflection may be very different this time. Chances are, there are lines and creases on your forehead, crow's-feet around your eyes, maybe even some crevices on your cheeks and deep brackets around your mouth.

In our teens and twenties, when we smile, we tend to have just a few folds of soft, plump skin around the eyes and, of course, when the face is at rest, it's completely smooth. But by the time we reach our late thirties, those little folds of soft skin may have turned into sharp-edged lines around the eyes. At this point our face can still look very youthful when it's motionless. However, once we enter our forties, most of us develop lines around the eyes that remain visible even when our faces are still. It's usually at about this age that many of us stop smiling into the mirror. Consciously or unconsciously, we start to avoid studying too closely the face that looks back at us. Have you noticed this about yourself?

You may find it interesting to know that muscles do not generate wrinkles anywhere on the body except on the face. Our facial muscles are unique. While other muscles originate on bone, then connect to bone, facilitating our ability to move, our facial muscles originate on bone but then attach directly to the skin. Therefore, every time you smile or frown the muscle pulls on the skin from underneath, making a wrinkle. When the skin is young, it does not matter because it snaps right back. But as the skin ages and collagen breaks down, the skin will yield to the pulling force and develop a wrinkle along the pulling force of the muscle.

As we grow older, we lose fat from the central part of the face. It's one of the cruelest tricks of nature that as we grow older, fat settles in the midsection of the body, where we don't want it and have such difficulty getting rid of it, yet we lose fat from the central part of the face, where, for the sake of our appearance, we need it. It's the loss of fat under the eyes and in the cheeks that gives rise to a hollowed, aged look. The loss of fat creates the lines that run from the nose to the mouth, which are known as *nasolabial folds*. It's also the loss of fat on the back of our hands and feet that gives the look of protruding veins and tendons on these parts of the body as we grow older.

Few people realize that the skin is just one component of the wrinkle. There are wrinkles without the skin component. In our early thirties, lines around the eyes often only show when we smile. The skin resists the pull of the muscle for a while. But as the skin collagen begins to break down, as a result of sun exposure and other intrinsic skin aging factors, the muscle pull lines become permanently etched into the skin, which means that the wrinkle has acquired the skin component as well. This is why we have lines around our eyes even when not smiling once we reach our forties. Eventually, the wrinkle will acquire the fat/connective tissue loss component as well. By our fifties, we may acquire deep nasolabial folds. These lines were first only muscle based, then muscle and skin based, as lastly, muscle, skin, and fat-loss based as well.

So here's the take-home message: *To win the war against wrinkles, you have to treat not only the skin, but the underlying muscle layer and the loss of fat as well.* If you are treating only one of the three causes of wrinkle formation, you are addressing only part of the condition.

Why does the skin give in and yield to the constant pulling force of muscles of facial expression? Why can it resist at age twenty and give in at forty? This has to do with skin aging, aging for both *extrinsic* (external) and *intrinsic* (internal) reasons. Remember the theories of aging we talked about in chapter 2? They all play a part.

Free radicals seek to steal an electron from healthy, intact molecules. If they steal from a collagen molecule in the skin, eventually the collagen molecule will become more rigid and compromised in its function.

Glycation occurs when sugar molecules cross-link skin collagen, making it more rigid and less functional.

Mitochondrial compromise, hormonal decline, and telomerase function changes, just to mention the most important factors, all affect the skin.

However, in spite of the powerful pro-aging forces, the skin actually is remarkably resilient and would last a lot longer if it were not for the chief extrinsic reason: the sun.

I can't stress enough how important it is to avoid sun exposure for the sake of your skin. When comparing the internal (intrinsic) reasons of skin aging to the main external (extrinsic) reason, which is the sun, the sun steals the show. It is by far the most significant reason why skin ages. Chances are that nearly everything you do not like about your skin ultimately comes from the sun.

You may say, "Oh, I hardly ever go in the sun." But you do not have to go "in the sun" for the sun to find you. Walk through a parking lot and you are sunning yourself; walk from the dry cleaner to the super-market and the sun finds you. Even five minutes of sun are too much. Sitting in the shade on your deck and having lunch is sun exposure. UV rays come through windows. Some halogen lights have UV rays.

What does the sun do to our skin?

The sun mercilessly breaks down collagen. Collagen is responsible for the elasticity of the skin, so as you lose collagen, the skin thins and becomes less elastic. As the muscle underneath pulls the skin, the skin develops wrinkles along the lines of facial expression. It also starts to sag along the jawline. Then, as the skin continues to thin and becomes more rigid, pores enlarge, red capillaries begin to show, and age and sun spots begin to appear. Skin cancers are beyond the scope of this book and I won't be discussing them, but they are the most dreaded consequences of sun exposure.

If you ever lose sight of why you have to protect your skin at all times, take a trip to a tropical location. Go on the beach and make friends with a woman from a previous generation, when ladies still sunned themselves. Take a look at the skin on her face. Compare it to skin somewhere on her body that has not been exposed to the sun. The two skin patches will look like they do not belong to the same person.

How *do* we treat wrinkles? It stands to reason that since there are three components to a wrinkle, we have to use a three-pronged ap-proach, addressing each factor separately.

THE SKIN COMPONENT OF A WRINKLE

In chapter 4 I describe how skin care has to be broken down into two phases: the skin-stimulating and -building step and the skin-sealing step. In the skin-stimulating/building step, the objective is to stimulate the skin's own collagen-making machinery, to build as much collagen as possible to thicken the appearance of the skin. This is the first step you can take on your own, at home, in the battle against wrinkles. Scientifically advanced skin care is an opportunity for you to improve your skin as never before, thanks to the recent development of ingredients that really work. Every day you can protect your skin from harmful sun rays and help control the damage created by free radicals, glycation, and other factors of aging.

Improving the appearance of the skin component of the wrinkle starts with daily exfoliation—there is no substitute for it for keeping the skin clear and radiant—followed by the use of thin, highly penetrating serums with key ingredients that deliver skin-stimulating and antioxidant ingredients.

As we've discussed before, skin becomes progressively thinner as we grow older; it's part of the natural aging process. For a woman, this process becomes exacerbated at menopause, with the dramatic drop in estrogen levels. The effect of the loss of this hormone is profound: the skin thins, lines develop, and elasticity diminishes rapidly. So the older a woman becomes, the more she can benefit from my six-step program, and the more she can benefit from understanding the key message I want to convey: *If you have lines and wrinkles on your face, "feel good" skin care will do very little for you; it will not build the skin the way you need.*

Aside from at-home skin-building care, there are several other medical-office based means available that will improve collagen production, thicken the skin, and reduce lines and wrinkles. These are skin rejuvenating and resurfacing procedures that involve polishing away dead skin cells from the top layer of skin (the epidermis) and/or removing the deeper, underlying layers (the dermis) to encourage the regeneration of fresh new skin. These treatments are generally referred to as "peels."

PEELS: TREATING THE SKIN COMPONENT OF A WRINKLE

When you hear the word "peel," you may associate it with a peel-off mask that cosmeticians used to give and sometimes even give today: some sort of rubbery or clay substance that solidifies on your face and peels off at the end of the session.

Lately the word "peel" has acquired a very different connotation. Now it refers to taking off various layers of skin. It means peeling the skin to various depths. Of course, in skin peels, *depth* is everything. It determines the results, the recovery time (if any), possible complications, and how many years it can take off your face (if any).

Peels can be sorted by depth, as in how much skin they remove.

- cosmetic exfoliation peels, which you would buy and administer for yourself

- superficial medical-office and spa-based peels

- medium-depth medical-office peels

- deep medical-office peels

Peels also can be sorted by the method of administration:

- Chemical peels. These use a variety of acids, such as glycolic, salicylic, and trichloric, at various strengths to strip away layers of skin.

- Mechanical peels. These include scrubs, the very popular *microdermabrasion* that uses a machine to emit a fine spray of salt, aluminum or magnesium crystals through a tube to polish away skin cells, as well as the much more invasive and risky medical dermabrasion that uses a spinning brush. (Medical dermabrasion is rarely performed these days except to remove deep-pitted acne scars.)

- Laser peels. These use laser energy to evaporate layers of skin.

Chemical peels can be over-the-counter (e.g., glycolic peel pads, vitamin C masks, AHA/BHA peel kits), superficial (in-office glycolic or salicylic peels), or medium or deep (performed with anesthesia by a doctor with a week or several weeks of recovery).

Mechanical peels can be over-the-counter (microdermabrasion creams), superficial (in-office microdermabrasion), or medium or deep (dermabrasion procedures performed by a doctor with anesthesia with weeks of recovery involved).

Laser peels can be superficial (in-office "laser facial" with no recovery time), medium or deep (laser peels performed by a doctor while you are under anesthesia—usually requires weeks of recovery).

What matters is not so much what method is used, but the depth of penetration, because depth determines the outcome and the recovery time involved.

How to Use Cosmetic Exfoliating Peels

Cosmetic exfoliating peels that you purchase for home use come in at least three varieties: chemical, mechanical (microdermabrasion creams), and enzymatic peels. What all of these different peels have in common is that they do not peel the skin to any dangerous degree. Nothing irreversible can happen to your skin, there is only an upside potential as long as you follow the directions and apply some common sense. There is such a wide margin of safety built into all these cosmetic peels that you do not have to worry: It is nearly impossible to get hurt as long as you follow the directions on the bottle. When a vendor puts a cosmetic peel on the market, the peel is diluted, mostly for fear of law-suits. In fact, the problem is that it is a bit too harmless. In any event, it still benefits you to some degree and, again, you are the best judge. If you see a change, great! Keep on using it. If you see no change, it is not your fault. The peel is not good enough.

Chemically based cosmetic peels for home use. These come in three main varieties: AHA or BHA peels or a combined AHA/BHA version. AHA means alpha-hydroxy acid, a supercategory that includes, among others, glycolic, lactic, and malic acids (from apples) and all the ones referred to colloquially as "fruit acids." The main BHA is salicylic acid (the same acid as in aspirin). Try to find a doctor's brand of home peel if possible. They are usually more powerful than the ones from a main-stream cosmetics house. I personally like Dr. Gross's Alpha-Beta Daily Face Peel (2%); it's not very strong because it is for everyday use, and it might be right for someone who has never used a peel before. DDF has a weekly AHA/BHA peel called Radiance 7-Day Peel kit that I like a lot. I've also heard good things about Dr. Murad's Vitamin C In-fusion Home Facial Kit. I have a rather strongly weekly peel called Dr. Denese's Triple Acid AHA/BHA Weekly Peel and a combined AHA/BHA 30 percent Vitamin C Tightening Mask that has a huge following.

These peels do make a significant difference in the skin. With reg-ular use, they exfoliate aggressively and they can soften the look of lines. They can also deep-clean pores and bring back radiance that you thought was long gone. If they do none of the above, move on. Find a stronger one.

Microdermabrasion home use creams. There is a remarkable upsurge of these creams on the market today. All the major cosmetics houses have one, and most doctors' lines have one. Trust your instincts. If you see a change in your skin, it is good cream. If you do not, move on. Again, doctors' lines usually carry stronger creams, but try a few. If it seems not to make a difference in your skin, return them. You know best. A good cream does not dry out the skin. I put ceramides (skin-identical lipids) in my microdermabrasion cream to replenish what lipids you lose during the course of abrasion. Do not worry if you lose lipids from the skin; they can be replenished fairly easily.

I do not recommend spending money on handheld microdermabrasion machines. Your hands do a much better job. You have more control—you can press harder and achieve better results.

Enzymatic home care peels. These contain enzymes, proteins that, in this context, are meant to "digest" old dead skin cells from the surface. This sounds menacing, I know, but it is harmless. In fact, this is perhaps the least effective way to exfoliate. But if it works for you, stick with it.

Keep using your home care peels regularly. Do not miss the chance to improve your skin. Use them several times a week; you can alternate between chemical and mechanical ones. Just remember: You can never exfoliate too much as long as you follow the directions on the bottle and apply some common sense. Also, keep using your daily glycolic peel pads, because this is the workhorse for your skin.

If you have the opportunity, go to a spa or a doctor's office for superficial peels as well. If you do not have the time or the finances, do not feel left out. But be even more serious about your daily glycolic peel pads and your weekly at-home peels and you will achieve results close to what a high-priced series of in-office doctor's peels can give you. To be honest, I have so little time, I seldom do in-office peels on myself. When I am in the office, I work on the faces of others, not on my own. But I've never missed a single day of my glycolic pads in the seven years that I've been making the products. I often use two a night, and I do a microderm peel and an AHA/BHA peel, with or without vitamin C, several times a week. Everyone tells me that I do not look my age.

Medical Office Peels

There are three categories of medical office peels: superficial (light), medium, and deep. Let's take a close look at each of them.

Superficial peels. Light peels or lunchtime peels are very popular, and for good reasons. Light peels, by definition, involve no recovery time.

The most popular ones are glycolic or salicylic acid peels or a micro-dermabrasion procedure. There are some laser procedures for superficial peels; however, they are expensive, and they don't give you much more than the light chemical peels. Even if a peel is performed by a laser, what counts is how deep it goes. A light peel never passes beyond the first layer of skin, the epidermis. It's sometimes even called a "lunchtime peel" because it can be done in an hour, and you can go back to work immediately.

A light peel will give you great exfoliation and cleaner pores, help improve whiteheads and blackheads, and, more importantly, help prevent their recurrence. It will rapidly bring radiance back to dull, ashen-looking skin, by taking off dead skin cells. And because it helps moisture reach the skin more effectively, a light peel will bring some changes in the look of lines, since the skin will be softer and more moisturized. However, light peel pads are unsafe to use for removal of wrinkles or discolorations. They simply do not go deep enough.

Medium-depth medical peels. Medium peels are more effective than superficial peels in improving the look of wrinkles, since the depth of the treatment reaches far enough to renew the top layer of skin after recovery. Medium-depth peels can be chemical, mechanical, or performed with a laser. Recovery time runs about five to eight days. They are most effective in treating the dark discoloration (age spots) that appears in skin as we grow older. But they're also helpful with lines and wrinkles. I will be discussing age spots and other signs of aging in detail in the next chapter.

A medium peel is usually administered under anesthesia (although, on occasion, pain medication may suffice). Only a doctor should perform a medium peel. Since both the epidermal and dermal layers of skin are involved, there are risks of permanent dark discolorations or white discolorations from loss of pigment, and even scars.

Salon and spa estheticians may not, by law, provide any services that would go as deep as a medium peel. These professionals offer many complicated, multistep cosmetic procedures, including facials, masks, microdermabrasion, light acid peels, and other skin exfoliating and moisturizing treatments. While the treatments may all feel good and be relaxing, none of these can compare to the results of a medium- or a superficial-depth peel performed by a physician in a medical office. Estheticians by law are prohibited from providing the stronger versions of superficial peels that a doctor is allowed to perform.

If an esthetician tells you that he or she can permanently improve your wrinkles, run, because any procedure he or she can legally provide simply cannot go deep enough into the skin to accomplish a permanent change in wrinkles or skin discoloration. To achieve significant collagen stimulation, the dermis layer must be reached, and this cannot happen with superficial peels.

Another caution: Don't let any salon or spa esthetician tell you that he or she can remove dark spots with light chemical peels or microdermabrasion. Nonmedical personnel cannot perform peels deep enough to remove dark spots. I see many salons advertising microdermabrasion or lunchtime glycolic, alpha-hydroxy or fruit acid peels as something that "removes lines and takes away dark skin discolorations." This is impossible, since microdermabrasion simply does not go deep enough to reach the color pigment layer of the skin. If it did, it would be called *macro*dermabrasion and it would have to be done under anesthesia, would cause bleeding, and would require a recovery time of at least a week. Nonmedical personnel are never qualified to administer such a procedure.

Deep medical peels. Deep peels are much like having a new lease on life for your skin. Your old skin will literally be burned off, but it will regenerate and be as smooth and flawless as the skin of a child. Deep peels can be chemical, mechanical, or performed by laser. These days, however, most deep peels are laser procedures, since this tool offers the most control. Deep peels are always performed under anesthesia. Deep peels, whether chemical, laser, or mechanical, reach the dermal layer of the skin. They have the most potential to regenerate collagen and truly remove lines and wrinkles.

The initial recovery time for deep peels can take up to fourteen to twenty-one days. By that I mean that during this period, you cannot go out of the house at all, because you will look positively frightening, even to yourself. I know burning off the facial skin sounds very scary, but it hurts very little, especially after the first day. However, make no mistake: The skin is open for many days. Redness can last up to six months, doctors often understate the amount of time it takes for the redness to disappear. Most patients can return to normal life within two to three weeks (thanks to the camouflaging properties of green makeup, which works well to cover and neutralize redness).

Deep peels are not for everyone. Very few people have them done, and it is usually a once-in-a-lifetime occurrence. You must be truly motivated and able to take in stride the emotional and physical challenges of such an invasive treatment.

You may ask, "Who in her right mind would go through a deep peel? What can possibly be the payoff?" You are right to wonder; there has to be a payoff, and it better be very significant, given what is involved.

Fortunately, the payoff *is extraordinary*. Lines and wrinkles disappear to a large extent, and pores shrink profoundly. The bad news is that anyone who has had a deep peel will *never* again be able to tan because most of the skin pigments in the face have been removed and will not regenerate. However, the skin itself always regenerates, unless the doctor went too deep, in which case it regenerates with scars. Fortunately, this tragic outcome is very rare, but this is why it's important to always be sure your doctor is qualified and experienced. Never allow anyone except a doctor to perform a deep peel on you. And I don't recommend traveling out of the country to have it done, either. There is too much at stake. In the United States, doctors are bound by strict laws and regulations. In foreign countries these regulations are often much looser.

Interestingly enough, the cells that regenerate the skin of the face are hiding deep down, in hair follicles that are submerged within the face. It is these deep tubular structures that survive the laser attack and provide the remarkable, essential function of producing the first new cells that then begin multiplying and dividing to repopulate the face with skin cells. The neck is never included in a deep peel because the skin will not regenerate properly. It would heal with scars. In fact, a deep peel cannot be done on any part of the body except the face.

Many celebrities choose to undergo deep peels. If you see a middle-aged celebrity in the press who has been stunningly rejuvenated, chances are that he or she not only had a face-lift, but also a deep skin peel.

Sometimes I see advertisements for topical products or light home peel treatments that feature before-and-after photographs of a model who obviously has had a deep laser peel. Of course, the general public is not supposed to know this. However, the changes are unmistakable to the trained eye. It saddens me how the public is taken for a ride at times.

HER FACE WAS HER FORTUNE

At thirty-eight, J. J., a professional model, felt her career was sliding. She was getting fewer and fewer plum assignments. A light-skinned blonde with freckles, age spots, and significant lines around the eyes, she very much looked her age, which she could not afford to do. Although she used good skin care and had microdermabrasion treatments regularly, these regimens could not make up for the significant sun exposure she'd had early in her life.

She was very articulate and clear about what she wanted when she came to see me. "I'm looking for the most drastic solution science has to offer to rejuvenate my skin as much as possible," she said.

"Well, a deep peel will help you," I told her. "But it will cost you a lot of time. Your recovery will take weeks, and you'll never be able to go in the sun again. You won't be able to tan anymore; because tanning will bring out dark blotches in your skin."

"I don't care. Whatever it takes," she said.

J. J. had a deep chemical peel. After the resurfacing procedure, she needed two weeks of complete home confinement. Her face remained red for three more months, and she had to use heavy makeup to conceal the color whenever she went out.

Six months later I asked her: "Was it worth it?"

"It was the hardest thing I have ever done in my life," she said, "but now I look nearly a decade younger. All my freckles and age spots are gone, as if they never existed before. And, more importantly, the lines around my eyes have disappeared as well. It is truly a new beginning for my skin. It was the best decision I have ever made."

OTHER OPTIONS

There is another new, noninvasive laser procedure on the market today that is worth mentioning here for the sake of completeness.

This is a new laser for skin rejuvenation that is nonablative, meaning it won't burn the skin. It operates on the principle of the laser stimulating the skin at the deeper layers of the face, directly bypassing the epidermis, so there is no open wound and, therefore, no recovery time. It sounds quite good in theory, except for most people it does not help very much. It helps 15 to 25 percent of cases, while in the rest of the patients the results are insignificant.

You may read about this procedure in magazines and newspaper articles, since the companies that produce these laser machines hire top public relations firms to generate publicity. The cost of the treatments is high—because the machines are remarkably (and unreasonably) expensive—but I don't recommend these procedures for anyone on a budget. The promise of minimal recovery time is true, but the promise of a stunning dermal rejuvenation comparable to medium and deep laser peels is not true. The results are minimal with few exceptions of positive outcome.

There is also a radio-frequency procedure that works for a relatively small percentage of patients. For the majority, the results are modest. You have to really look for an improvement in wrinkles; any change is far from obvious. The risk to the skin is minimal, but the risk to your pocketbook is great. If you don't mind spending several thousand dollars on a procedure that may or may not work for you, go ahead. If your resources are limited, do it the hard, proven, and predictable way: Go through the extensive recovery time, because the good skin that comes from the regeneration process of a medium or deep peel is yours to keep forever.

BOTOX: TREATING THE MUSCLE COMPONENT OF A WRINKLE

All traditional topical skin care addresses only the skin, not the muscle or the fat component underneath. This is because, until recently, this was all that the industry knew how to do. But these days, doctors can combine resurfacing procedures with treatments that address the underlying muscles. Botox (botulinum toxin) injections are the most common and successful way to address the muscle layer.

Peels, of course, do nothing for the muscle layer. They treat the skin exclusively, by thickening it and increasing the health and the number of the collagen molecules, thereby making the skin thicker and more elastic. Once a peel has been performed and newly formed collagen grows in, wrinkles can be regenerated by the same muscle-pulling force that created them the first time around. So it pays to give the skin a rest by relaxing the underlying muscles with an injection of Botox after the peel has healed.

Botox was originally used to treat a condition called strabismus, commonly known as cross-eye. When it was seen that the injections flattened wrinkles around the eyes with a never before seen speed and efficacy, the treatments quickly spread into the area of cosmetic medicine. Botox brought about profound changes in skin care because, for the first time, dermatologists were able to see the remarkable impact of muscle pull in wrinkle formation. Botox treats lines on the forehead and around the eyes exceptionally well, visibly flattening them for three to six months by cutting back on the muscle's ability to contract and pull on the skin.

Botox is predominantly used in the forehead and around the eye area for crow's-feet. It is very rarely used on the lower part of the face and around the mouth, because it can easily result in an asymmetrical smile. No doctor wants to run the risk of leaving a patient with a crooked smile. It can be used in the neck to reduce the tendonness or "cording" look of the neck. It's an expensive procedure—a neck treatment can cost as much as $2,000 per session, and it has to be repeated every several months. Given the cost, few people can afford it.

Botox's side effects are rare. The most common, a slight drooping of one eyelid, lasts for a few weeks, then resolves by itself, without any known exceptions.

The injections hurt. It helps to ice the area beforehand or apply an anesthetic cream, which also reduces the development of black-and-blue marks at the injection site.

The price hurts even more: $400 to $600 per session. Botox is another sad case of a medication with an overinflated cost, resulting from the lack of price regulations in the pharmaceutical industry. I know many women who go into debt and who sacrifice on household expenses, food, and education to be able to afford it. Others, sadly, just feel left out.

"Will my face grow expressionless from Botox?" is a question I frequently hear from new patients. This is a common misconception. I doubt that there are many actors over thirty in Hollywood who do *not* have Botox in their face at all times. And although the performing artists in Hollywood are sometimes more interested in looking pretty than expressing emotion, Botox won't prevent you from making a face if you want to.

Botox is not for every skin. It works wonders for anyone who is middle-aged, but by a certain age and wrinkle level, it becomes counter-productive. For those in their late sixties and seventies, it can produce the appearance of more wrinkles. In the elderly, Botox may actually cause the skin to bunch up under the eyes and create the look of bags and more wrinkles. Some doctors, all too eager to have your business, may not tell you this. Once again, I hope to help you to be prepared and to be careful.

THE TOPICAL ALTERNATIVE TO BOTOX

Let's face it: There is nothing that is more effective in treating the muscle component of a wrinkle than Botox. However, Botox may not be an option for everyone.

If you find it too expensive or you hate the idea of injections or pain, there is another way to go—a topical alternative. A new generation of scientifically advanced ingredients has been developed that claim to decrease the contractile force of the muscles around the eyes. According to company claims, the new ingredient, *Argireline,* is able to address not only the skin, but the underlying muscle layer (i.e., the movement-related component of the wrinkle) as well. There is very little scientific research on the ingredient and the effects are minimal compared to the injections, but it is worth a try.

Some of the most progressive cosmetics manufacturers, such as Lancôme, Avon, and Gatineau have come out with products that contain Argireline. Try Lancôme Resolution Wrinkle Concentrate D-Contraxol, Avon Anew Clinical Line & Wrinkle Corrector, Gatineau DefiLift 3D Face Tensor and DDF Wrinkle Relax.

I have also designed a serum that incorporates Argireline at its maximum recommended concentrations, called Zero Tox 2. In fact, as far as I know, I was the first to create such a product. Since I produce a small line of skin-care products, I am able to respond quickly to new research, and I don't have to consult a committee about the cost ingredients. It is my principle not to ask the cost of a raw ingredient until I have determined the best formula for maximum effectiveness because I do not want to be influenced by the price. The high price of the new medical Argireline makes it virtually unusable to "angel dusting."

Of course, whether or not the major cosmetics companies have put these ingredients into the jar in quantities that are significant enough to make the product effective can only be determined by you after you've tried the formula. In skin-care products, everything rises or falls on the raw ingredient percentages. Keep an open mind when using these products. *Expect* results. And if you do not get them, remind yourself that it is not your fault. It is the fault of the product. Maybe the company decided to spend more on advertising and less on the key ingredients. Be critical and keep looking for the product that delivers results for you. It is out there.

COLLAGEN AND RESTYLANE: TREATING THE FAT AND CONNECTIVE TISSUE COMPONENTS OF A WRINKLE

As we age, fat leaves the face and settles on our abdomen and buttocks, as so many of us know so well. As I've discussed before, when the face ages, the lines deepen, not only because of collagen loss in the skin and the repetitive pull of muscle movement, but also because of significant loss of subcutaneous fat.

What effect does fat loss have on the face? The lines from the bottom of the nose to the corner of the mouth (nasolabial folds) deepen; lines running down from the corner of the mouth (marionette lines) deepen; the eye area hollows out; the sides of the forehead become bony; and the fat over the cheekbones dissipates. These are the hallmarks of the aging face. Fat, our archenemy in every other area of the body, is sorely missed in the face as we grow older.

Unfortunately, this is a very difficult problem to solve. Truly, there is *no* good topical solution that can correct fat loss. *Any advertisements, any claims that promise a cream or a mask that will soften nasolabial folds or marionette lines, are a vast overstatement.* Do not be persuaded. These ads do exist. I have seen them. So beware.

The *only* way to treat the loss of fat in the face is with injectable fillers. They are used, predominantly, in the lower part of the face. The ideal place for them is in nasolabial folds and marionette lines. In these areas, fillers can make a remarkable difference to your appearance, taking years off the look of the face.

Fillers are *not* suitable for the eye area, where the skin is thin, and the filler tends to lump, causing surface irregularities and bumpiness. Fillers are also *not* suitable for filling out cheekbones and the hollowness around the eyes. Sometimes they cause lumpiness under the skin that gives the face a strange, synthetic look.

Some doctors are willing to inject fillers into the upper part of the face, often with very artificial-looking results. Be sure to go only to an experienced medical doctor for filler injections, and don't be afraid to ask if you can expect any lasting lumpiness under your skin as a result of the process. You might be surprised how often the answer could be yes. This will make the doctor realize that you know what you are talking about. A patient needs to be fully informed before undergoing any cosmetic procedure.

The best filler for the upper part of the face (under the eyes and at the cheekbones) is *your own fat*. Fat that has been drawn from your own body, then reinjected into the upper part of the face, can be remarkably successful because your own fat is thin, pliable, and distributes well under thin skin. Injecting the face with fat is a very delicate procedure, so again, be sure that you go to someone with experience.

There are a number of other injectable fillers on the market these days. The first to be used, more than a decade ago, were two types of highly purified bovine (cow) collagen. Now we know that collagen is one of the least desirable fillers because it does not last, for starters. Collagen must be tested for an allergic reaction. Doctors should test twice, to be safe, and even then collagen still may trigger an allergic reaction while inside your face. When this happens it is very bad news. If an allergic reaction occurs, with collagen that was injected in the nasolabial fold, the injection tract can remain bright red for many months. The condition will resolve eventually, but it is a long and rocky road for the patient.

Currently, hyaluronic acid fillers are being used most successfully. Hyaluronic acid is a fluid that exists naturally in all living organisms. In the human body it's found in the joints; in the fluid of the eyes; and, most abundantly, in the skin. The first hyaluronic filler to be approved in the United States is Restyline. It has no allergic potential, distributes well, and can last for up to four to five months. It is ideal in the nasolabial folds or marionette lines. But if you're considering having it injected into the upper part of the face, I'd advise you to proceed with great caution and do your homework on your doctor. Bumpiness can easily develop under the eyes or on the cheekbones, and it may not go away. Pearline is another filler on the market that is in the family of hyaluronic acids. It can last in the face for up to a year.

HAPPY ENDINGS

As you see, to wage a campaign against wrinkles, the battles must be fought on three fronts. For the skin, there are topical products and peels. For the muscles, there is Botox and a few promising ingredients that may also address the muscles topically. For the loss of fat, there are fillers. These alternatives run the spectrum from gentle and noninvasive to extreme resurfacing with long recovery times. The good news about all of them is that they work. You can choose what is most appropriate for your needs and your pocketbook. By combining the right treatments for your specific needs with my daily program and with healthy habits for living, you can have beautiful, younger-looking skin for life.

DOCTOR'S OFFICE VS. SPA

Many people ask me "Should I go to a facialist regularly for cleansing facials, or should I go to a doctor's office for superficial peels?"

Believe me, I have many more patients than I ever could or want to see, so I am not looking for business. My commitment is to *you* and not to building my practice. The practice builds by itself as long as I take care of you the way it should be done.

Choosing between regular facials and light peels from a doctor's office, or a doctor-supervised medical spa, is a choice between your skin *looking good* versus *feeling good*. It is that simple.

Facialists steam your face and try to clean your pores by messing with them one by one. The chance of infection under these conditions is very high. It is far easier and more effective to "unroof" the whiteheads and blackheads first, then let them spill their contents on their own. This is what superficial chemical or mechanical peels (microdermabrasion) will do for you.

There are many spas that offer light chemical peels and microdermabrasion these days. You have to realize that spas are very limited in terms of the effectiveness of these procedures. They are limited *by law* as to the strength of the light chemical peels, and also they are not allowed, *by law,* to purchase the same-strength microdermabrasion machinery as doctors or doctor-supervised medical spas. Lasers for noninvasive "laser facials" are another case in point. Some spas list laser facials on their service menu. Believe me, the kind of "laser facial" that a medically unsupervised facialist can perform is so light that it borders on the ineffective.

Many complicated multistep facial procedures with fancy names are available at spas these days. They make you feel good and cared for, and there is a place for that. However, the results are minimal and entirely temporary.

Medical spas are very different. Be careful; there are many spas that call themselves medical spas. They consider themselves medispas because they know the physician around the corner, or one of the facialists worked as a nurse's aide one summer. I am exaggerating, but you get the point. The only spas that can be called medical spas have to have a physician on the premises to directly supervise what is taking place. A loose affiliation—"I know Dr. X, we send him patients, so we can say that he is our supervising physician"—is *not good enough.* You will not get strong and effective treatments without a physician involved. You are paying top dollar, so you should get the benefits.

CHAPTER SIX

THE SIGNS OF AGING

Time to look in the mirror again. Don't look for wrinkles this time, look for the seven other signs of aging of the skin. Look particularly at the T-zone (the area around the nose and cheeks). Do you see enlarged pores and bumpiness under the skin? Do you see redness? Are there dark spots that weren't there a few years ago? Does your skin seem dull and sallow? Does it feel dry and thin? Does your face sag around the jawline and under the chin?

Chances are, unless you are still in your early twenties, you'll see some of these signs of aging. That's the bad news. The good news is that it's not too late to deal with these problems. Let's take them one by one.

ENLARGED PORES

More bad news, I'm afraid. Our pores enlarge throughout our lives. If you think it's bad now, it will only get worse. This skin condition doesn't stop its downward spiral until late in life, at which point, in the context of all the problems of an aging complexion, it becomes minor.

Remember the three components of a wrinkle—skin, underlying muscle, and subcutaneous fat and connective tissue? The enlarged pore has only one responsible party: the skin itself. The underlying muscle layer is not involved, and the subcutaneous fat and connective tissue losses play no part. This is good news, because it means that if the skin can be rejuvenated, the pores can be improved.

Pores enlarge for the same reasons that skin develops wrinkles: loss of collagen, loss of elasticity, and thinning of the skin. As a result of the lack of elasticity, the skin grows less able to close the pores. It's as simple as that.

Yet enlarged pores is not a problem for everyone. I often see women the same age, with the same level of skin aging, and yet one has enlarged pores and the other does not. Why? Thick and oily skin is more prone to enlarged pores in the T-zone because oil and debris on the skin may increase pore size. If you have oily skin, the benefit is that you will develop fewer lines and wrinkles as you age than someone with thin, less porous skin. You may have enlarged pores, but she will have lines sooner than you. Everything comes with a price.

If you have thin, dry-to-normal skin, enlarged pores aren't likely to become an issue until you reach your forties or fifties, when a significant amount of collagen may break down due to aging and sun exposure.

Yes, sun exposure is another major contributor to enlarged pores. Many of my patients are surprised when I mention the sun as a factor in enlarging pores. They know that the sun will give them spots and lines, but enlarged pores? The truth is, one good tan in the summer will lead to more visible pores the following winter. The origin of pores and lines is virtually identical. Everything that ages the skin applies to pores in the same way.

So what can be done for the problem?

One of the most important things you can do for your pores is to clean them throughly every night. Of course, all of us fully intend to clean our face every night. We line up our cleanser and toner and start cleansing. But as I explained in my six-step program, washing with a good cleanser is an excellent start, but not enough. Next, you'll need to wipe your face with a cotton ball soaked in a toner. You will be surprised how much dirt it picks up. Both the cleanser and the toner should contain glycolic acid (alpha-hydroxy and/or beta-hydroxy acids), which actually dissolves the "glue" that holds the skin cells together, so surface cells dislodge and slide off. Commercial glycolic acid cleansers (even expensive ones) will not be sufficient. Typically a glycolic acid cleanser contains 1 to 2 percent glycolic acid. This is not strong enough.

Since, throughout the day, your pores collect sebum (semifluid secretions from the subcutaneous glands) and debris, encouraging them to grow ever larger, you need some high technology in addition to cleanser and toner. You need an agent that can dissolve sebum and dislodge old dead skin cells that clog the pores. Glycolic acid, fruit acids, and salicylic acid are the best choices. My recommendation is that, after cleansing and toning at night, you use a high-percentage acid peel pad to deep clean pores and exfoliate. Remember, this is not a "feel good" product. It should tingle as you clean the face. However, a properly acidic, pH-balanced pad should *not* leave your face feeling dry when you finish. In fact, your skin should feel fresh, clean, and moisturized. If it feels dry, it's not your fault. It's the fault of the pad. Get rid of it.

After these three steps, you can rest assured that your pores are as clean as modern science can make them.

THE SIGNS OF AGING | 99

THE POWER OF PADS

Thirty-five-year-old Maria was of Italian descent, with thick skin that was especially oily in the T-zone. She was concerned about the pores on her face. They were enlarged all around her nose and cheeks, distributed in the pattern of a butterfly. She came to me ready to do whatever it might take to make them disappear.

I explained to her that the most important thing she could do was to clean her face thoroughly every night, with cleanser, toner, and a glycolic acid pad. If she neglected any step in the process, sebum and dirt would settle in her pores, gradually enlarging them further before their time, and the formation of blackheads and whiteheads would be a pressing issue as well. As a last step, I recommended a thin, penetrating serum loaded with antioxidants.

Four weeks later, Maria returned for more products and to tell me that for the first time ever, her pores appeared to be and her blackheads had improved remarkably. She said she couldn't imagine ever skipping a day with her three-step cleansing process, especially the pads.

"Without the pads," she said, "my skin just doesn't feel clean."

If you have normal to oily skin and are troubled by enlarged pores, use a microdermabrasion cream several times a week in addition to the three cleaning steps. You are the best judge of how many times per week are right for you—but certainly no fewer than twice a week. Additional mechanical abrasion can only facilitate the cleaning process. You may benefit from regular, in-office superficial peels. Please, avoid "feel good" facials at spas. Look for serious superficial glycolic or salicylic acid treatments combined with microdermabrasion (usually found in a doctor's office). The idea is to undergo the most extensive exfoliating treatment you can without incurring any recovery time.

The next step in pore care is skin rejuvenation to help facilitate the skin's collagen-making machinery, which, as I've explained, is what pulls the pores together. As I've recommended before, this is best done with a thin, penetrating serum loaded with antioxidants such as carnosine, vitamins, and collagen-stimulating amino acid peptides in a glycolic acid base.

It is also important *not* to use a cream on an oily T-zone. Moisture is not an issue for an oily area, and if you feed it with an oily cream, it may clog pores. However, you do need to use a lipid-based moisturizing serum around the eye area. This region never seems to have enough oil, even if the rest of the face is oily.

When I first opened my practice and began to see patients with skin concerns, I was stunned by how often enlarged pores headed the list of complaints. One forty-six-year-old woman who came to see me, with thin, dry, very light-colored skin, told me that her chief concern was her pores. I was surprised and waited for her list of complaints to continue, because I saw at least three other areas on her face—dark discolorations, lines, and a loosening jawline—that I thought were far more significant to making her look her age. But it turned out the pores were all that troubled her. Then she told me that her eyesight had changed recently, so she'd bought a new magnifying mirror and realized, for the first time, that her pores were a big problem. I reminded her that people don't carry magnifying mirrors around to look at your face. And that's a good thing!

CLOGGED PORES AND BUMPINESS UNDER THE SKIN

Clogged pores and bumpiness under the skin are caused by sebaceous products that get stuck under the skin. Since they have nowhere to go, they form bumps—most often on the forehead and around the nose. Often this condition is the direct result of inappropriate skin care.

A case in point: Sarah, a twenty-seven-year-old financial manager, came to me obsessing over the clogged pores and small bumps on her forehead, nose, and cheeks. She had normal skin, with a bit of excess oiliness on the T-zone.

Given her age, I was surprised to see the unevenness of Sarah's skin surface. Usually, in youth, the skin is tight and straight and only loosens and acquires an uneven texture later. I suspected at once that Sarah's problem might be self-induced. So the first questions I asked her were about her daily skin-care routine.

She used a creamy cleanser every day, she told me, along with a thick, famous, expensive, rich night cream. The perfect regimen for someone *fifty years her senior*! I asked her what possessed her to use a cleanser and cream more suited for her grandmother. She told me, "These products are so expensive—I figured they had to be good!"

I understood Sarah. We are all so caught up trying to look young. An expensive cream with a big promise is hard to resist. But remember: The skin does not like to be choked. Creams choke the skin.

Now, thanks to skin-care science, we know that choking the skin belongs in the past. The primary purpose of creams is to cover the skin and prevent water loss. In terms of getting the key ingredients to permeate the skin, the cream is not the best vehicle because sometimes the very moisturizing particles that make the cream feel good on the skin can stand in the way of the ingredients' penetration. A thin serum is better suited to deliver active ingredients.

Rather than being suffocated with heavy cream, the skin wants to breathe, which is why you must exfoliate. And you can't exfoliate too much; whatever you take off comes back, amply. The skin needs to be stimulated by various acids, high-potency vitamins, peptides—and only then be given some skin-identical lipids to seal it all.

I told Sarah to give her expensive jar of cream to her grandmother—that oily, rich product was really best suited for dry, older skin. Then

I jump-started Sarah's skin care with a series of combination chemical and microdermabrasion peels to aggressively exfoliate and clear her pores.

Her home care was just as important as the office treatments, and her new regime began with the three-step cleansing system: cleanser, toner, and a high-percentage glycolic pad every night, followed by a thin serum with a high percentage of key ingredients, including carnosine, vitamins, antioxidants, AHA/BHA, and amino acid peptides. She also used a microdermabrasion cream twice a week. She no longer put any cream on her T-zone. In fact, she only used cream around her eyes. Within a few weeks, her skin cleared up; the bumpiness, blackheads, and whiteheads disappeared; and she began to look twenty-seven again.

Fortunately, whatever pore clogging or bumpiness you may have created by the inappropriate use of products can be reversed, too, to some extent.

WHAT ABOUT FACIALS?

I'm often asked by patients who suffer from clogged pores and skin bumpiness if they should get a cleansing facial—the traditional kind, in which the face is first steamed, and then clogged pores are emptied by extraction, one by one.

This process has been handed down from generation to generation, when there was truly nothing else that could be done to cleanse the pores. The problem with it has always been that it is impossible to do a really good job. The pores will not completely clear just because the skin has been steamed a bit. Skin is thick, and it would take a lot more than steaming to achieve this end. Also, how can you clean all of the pores?

All this process really results in is redness; more bumps; and, sometimes, even breakouts.

In my office, I no longer allow the estheticians to do a steam cleaning without a pretreatment. First, we do an acid peel combined with an aggressive microdermabrasion procedure. We loosen the "glue" between the surface cells with the acid; then we abrade the skin, taking off some of the epidermis.

If the skin is opened up in this way, the sebaceous material that is the substance of the bumps may find its way to the surface by itself. And many more pores will clear than can be emptied in the traditional one-by-one approach.

I find that the combination of a light chemical and mechanical peel works well to even out the bumpiness of the skin surface, although it does take a few sessions.

SALLOW SKIN

Sallow skin usually comes late in life. When we're in our twenties and thirties, our skin exfoliates well even by itself, giving us the pinkish, radiant glow of new skin cells. Then comes a time when exfoliation becomes very sluggish. The glow is lost; the radiant, pinkish overtone of new skin is gone. Dry, old cells begin to occupy the skin surface; hence the color change we call ashen, dull, or sallow.

The good news is that under every dull complexion, there is a layer of youthful new skin. The one thing we do *not* have to give up as we grow older is skin color. All it takes to maintain it is an understanding of how the skin works and an open mind.

My patient Karen was forty-nine years old when she came to see me for the first time. She had a lot of sun exposure in her history—she'd just moved to New York from California, where she'd lived most of her life—and her skin was thin, dry, and very dull-looking. She'd been treating it for many years as if it were as delicate as cigarette paper, using a rich, creamy cleanser. Sometimes she wouldn't wash her face with water—just tissue it off with the cleanser. And—you guessed it—she used a rich cream day and night.

I recommended a combination of a light chemical peel with microdermabrasion. At first she was very afraid—such a treatment went against all her long-held beliefs about how her delicate skin should be pampered. I explained that the primary benefit of superficial peels is to solve the radiance problem. Superficial peels take off just enough skin so no time is needed for recovery, but the fresh new skin cells underneath the old dead ones can be liberated. I was so convinced that Karen would benefit from the exfoliation, and so reluctant to see her miss out on better-looking skin because of misplaced fear, that I told her she wouldn't have to pay for the treatment unless she liked the outcome. It was an offer she couldn't resist. She loved the results so much that she signed up for a series of peels, and she hasn't missed a month for the past two years.

Fortunately, the problem of sallow skin can be solved at home with results that are comparable to what can be provided by superficial peels in a doctor's office. I remember when I came to this country, with only $40 in my pocket. I wasn't able to take care of my skin properly—I just couldn't afford to. But today, thanks to new products, you don't need a lot of money to take care of your skin. If you live in an area where doctors' lunchtime peels are not available just around the corner, or you would rather save your money to put your kids through college, do not despair. The benefit of superficial peels can be yours, done at home and at a reasonable cost.

With my program, you clean and tone at night, then use a glycolic pad to exfoliate. Initially, simply pat your face gently with the pad. Then, as you get used to it and your tolerance increases, rub more aggressively. Follow this step by applying a glycolic-based serum with a high percentage of all the beneficial key ingredients that I've mentioned throughout this book. Also use a microdermabrasion cream. Start with once a week; then, as your tolerance grows, up the usage to two to three times a week.

There are some doctor-designed AHA/BHA peels (DDF Radiance 7-Day Peel Kit, Dr. Gross's Alpha-Beta Daily Face Peel, and my own Facial Firming pads and Triple Acid AHA/BHA Weekly Peel, to name a few) that are excellent for weekly use, in addition to all the above. Prescription Retin A and Renova are also very good choices, although be warned: I know very few adults who can use them daily. If you can build up a tolerance for them, I am happy for you, but it will likely be a long, rocky road for your skin to get accustomed.

Here's a tip: Retin A and Renova become more irritating when mixed with water, so if you use a prescription Retin A, wait at least twenty minutes after you wash your face to allow the water in your skin to evaporate; then apply the Retin A. And remember, if you are on prescription-strength Retin A, use the glycolic pads and acidic serums with great care, and stop if your skin gets irritated.

Retinol is chemically related to tretinoin, which is the key ingredient in prescription-strength Retin A and Renova.

Retinol is present in non-prescription cosmetic products but it is not as effective as Retin A and Renova. Retinol is a very expensive ingredient (about $3,000 per kilogram). As a point of comparison, most ingredients are more in the range of $80 to $150 per kilogram. Cosmetics industry executives tend to find the price of retinol very high and the product can be irritating to the skin; therefore, cosmetics companies keep the percentage in their products down to a symbolic amount. Keep this in mind when you see the claims the product makes. And remember, you know better than anyone what works for your skin.

My final advice on sallow skin: You cannot overexfoliate as long as you follow the directions and apply common sense. All you have to lose is a dull complexion.

DARK DISCOLORATION OF THE SKIN

Sadly, the problem of dark discoloration is the area of skin care in which cosmetics companies are most likely to take you for a ride.

How many of you bought a skin-care product that promises a

skin-lightening, skin-brightening, or skin-fading effect, only to find that it does not work at all? You start to use it, it does not seem to do much, then you lose interest and use it less and less. After a while you stop using it and conclude that it did not work probably because you did not have the discipline to use it consistently. You think it's your fault.

Interestingly enough, this time it's not entirely the fault of the cosmetics companies. Let me explain.

In the field of dermatology, skin discoloration is one of the most difficult conditions to solve. The medically sanctioned ingredient to tackle the problem is called *hydroquinone*. It works by inhibiting the manufacture of new pigment cells. However, it doesn't do anything for dark spots once they've appeared. Pigment cells have about a six-week life span, after which they break down and are replaced by new cells. So if hydroquinone is prescribed, and the formation of some of the new pigment cells is inhibited, dark spots may fade from your complexion over time. The typical prescription dose of hydroquinone is 4 percent, but even at that strength it is only moderately effective. Sometimes, combined with glycolic acid, its effectiveness improves a bit, but I have yet to speak with a patient who was completely satisfied with the outcome of any prescription fading cream.

So why, you may ask, isn't hydroquinone prescribed in a higher strength?

The answer is that if the percentage is increased it becomes very irritating. It's a classic case of damned if you do, damned if you don't.

Hydroquinone, by law, cannot be sold over-the-counter in more than 2 percent strength. So you see, if it works only moderately at 4 percent strength, it's no wonder that the high-priced department store brand creams with only half the power are not effective. This time, as I said, the cosmetics industry can't be held entirely at fault.

Here's the take-home message: If dark spots trouble you, don't waste your money in a department store, and definitely don't waste your time on light chemical peels and microdermabrasion in spas, because you will invariably be disappointed. Superficial peels don't work well because the color pigments are too deep for the acids or microdermabrasion to reach. Please, do not let anyone mislead you into thinking they can remove dark spots by superficial means.

There *are* spot treatments for dark discolorations with lasers. The laser energy selectively burns the dark skin patches, turning them even darker temporarily. Then they peel off. The process should work after one session. If it doesn't, don't go back—and don't let anyone tell you that you need to return several times.

There are some botanical skin-fading agents, unregulated by the FDA, that come to the rescue in over-the-counter products. And a few serums, not creams, deliver these ingredients with some success.

SkinCeuticals PhytoCorrective Gel fading serum, developed by a famous Egyptian chemist, Dr. Omar, performs well. My line also includes a fading serum of which I am very proud. The key ingredient, arbutin, competes with the price of gold. So major cosmetics companies are not rushing to put this ingredient into their products. They have to answer to a higher authority—a bottom-line-conscious board of directors. Luckily, I do not.

One of the reasons why a fading cream doesn't work well is pretty simple. You put the cream on at night and it has a tendency to rub off on the pillow while you're sleeping. And if it's on the pillow, it will do no good for your skin. Try this experiment: put cream on your face at night and see if it's still there in the morning. I know mine is always gone from my face by the middle of the night, so I invented a skin patch that has the skin-fading ingredients built in. Put the patch on a spot, and it will stay all night, delivering ingredients directly to the discolored area.

There is also a very aggressive Retin A/hydroquinone prescription-strength treatment called the Obagi Nu-Derm System, developed by a Middle Eastern doctor, Zein Elabdine Obag. It rarely fails. I have seen hundreds of women who were significantly helped by it.

The catch is that for the first three weeks, your face will be red, dry, and peeling. You can go to work, but the irritation will be noticeable. It will seem that the lines around your eyes have deepened—an increase in dryness always creates that impression. I give my patients a lipid serum for the eye area, which makes a great difference. However, in four to six weeks with the Obagi System, there is a remarkable improvement in dark discolorations. Good things come to those who really try. If you can endure the treatment, you can reap great rewards, both in skin fading and skin tightening. The products are available online. Obagi Clear and Obagi Exfoderm Forte are especially effective.

If you are over forty and you haven't worn SPF sun protection daily for the past twenty years, even if you haven't spent much time on a beach, you may still have dark marks on your skin. A medium-depth peel (with an erbium laser or trichloric acid) may be an excellent solution to removing them. It can reach deep enough into the skin to mobilize pigment changes and can result in a perfectly even complexion. And skin without blotches, of course, will look much more youthful.

If you have black or brown skin, which is high in pigment (melanin), you may have dark marks as a result of acne, as well. With dark skin, even after acne clears up, spots remain, and medium-depth peels can remove them very effectively.

It's logical to suppose that thin, fair, Caucasian skin is fragile and less resilient to laser or acid peels than strong, thick, dark skin, but the opposite is true. Darker skins are more sensitive and vulnerable by far. Medium-depth peels are the *maximum*-depth peels that can be performed on individuals of Arab, African, Asian, Hispanic, Indian, and Native American descent. If you have dark skin, you need to be extremely careful. You should *never* go to anyone except an experienced medical doctor for skin peels or laser treatments because inexperienced, un-medically trained hands can leave permanent dark or light blotches on your skin.

A CAUTIONARY TALE: THE PEEL
THAT WENT TOO DEEP

At thirty-four, Angela, a beautiful African-American woman, came into my office with a skin disfigurement that couldn't be reversed. She had a prominent light-colored patch, surrounded by a very dark border, under one eye.

She'd had acne when she was a teenager, she told me. Every breakout had produced a dark spot that never seemed to fade and go away. By the time she was an adult, her face was covered with dark spots. She'd heard that a chemical peel could even out her skin tone, and she'd consulted a "skin-care professional," who, unfortunately, wasn't medically licensed or trained.

Angela was given a trichloric acid peel that left her with even darker discolorations in areas where the skin was peeled too deep. Even worse, in some places she lost pigment altogether, and once pigment is totally lost, it can never be replaced.

Angela had put herself into the wrong hands and now had to live with the consequences of that choice for the rest of her life. I've never forgotten her.

I'm telling her story here as a warning to others with dark skin, who should never be given a medium chemical or laser treatment by anyone except a doctor.

Cosmetic dermatology for dark skin is very special. Lines and wrinkles are less of a problem, but dark discolorations are a major issue. In fact, the mark of aging for dark skin is a progressive, often uneven and blotchy darkening, especially around the mouth. If mature dark skin is lightened and made more even-toned, it will look years younger.

Superficial and medium-depth peels can cause dark skin to turn even darker if the skin is overirritated, although this problem is reversible in most cases. The most successful way to treat the dark discolorations on ethnic skin is with the Obagi System. It is remarkably effective. If you have dark skin, I advise you *not* to let an esthetician sell you expensive lightening creams, since nothing that can be sold over-the-counter by the skin-care trade will be strong enough to really lighten your skin. Save your money for the prescription-strength Obagi System. It does the trick every time. The only times I've seen the Obagi System fail is when patients have skipped steps and ignored instructions.

RED CAPILLARIES

Visible red capillaries under the skin (a medical condition called *telangiectasia*) invariably get worse over time. They start around the nose and then invade the cheeks and the chin. The thinner the skin, the more likely it is to show red capillaries, especially if they are chronically dilated—and, unfortunately, chronic dilation is another frequent age-related occurrence.

Recently I received a phone call from a fifty-four-year-old woman named Sophia. Originally from Sweden, Sophia had lived most of her life in Florida, where she was a competitive swimmer. She began to tell me her primary skin concern, when I surprised her by interrupting and finishing her sentence for her. I didn't have to see her in person to know she had a problem with red capillaries.

Anyone who has light skin and who has had a lot of sun exposure can count on red capillaries later in life. The lighter the skin tone and hair color and the more sun exposure, the worse the problem will be. Menopause greatly hastens red capillaries as well, since after menopause, the skin thins even further.

Rosacea is often confused with telangiectasia. It's understandable, since rosacea presents with visible red capillaries, redness, and flushing (see chapter 8 for more on rosacea). However, rosacea has an inflammatory, acnelike, pustular component to it that telagiectasia does not, and it's important to get an accurate diagnosis, because the treatments are not the same.

If you suspect that you have telangiectasia or rosacea, you need to see a doctor. Don't let your hairdresser or your neighborhood facialist diagnose you.

Lasers are the treatment of choice for red capillaries. The lasers work by heating the blood in the capillary. When blood is heated, it coagulates, then breaks down in response. The blood vessel then clogs, and the remnants are absorbed into the body. You may be red and irritated from the laser treatment for a day, but that reaction will be gone by the next day.

If your visible capillaries are very red on a light background, this treatment can be successful. However, if your blood vessel is so light that you can only see it with your 3X magnifying mirror, don't bother seeking laser treatment. It won't do much, and no one is looking at your face with a magnifying mirror anyway!

Typically, the laser treatment needs to be repeated several times at first, and then you must go back for maintenance visits. The reason is because when one capillary closes, another often generates in its place. Dynamically, if the blood pressure conditions are such that the blood wants to flow that way, then that's the way it will flow, and the capillaries will show.

There are creams that claim to improve telangiectasia through various botanical extracts. However, in my experience, if there is any improvement, it will be minimal.

Hot weather, heated living conditions, and spicy foods all exacerbate telangiectasia, but sun damage is the fastest way to accelerate it. So use your sunscreen every day.

There is one lasting (albeit drastic) way to improve telangiectasia, and that's a deep peel. A deep peel works because it significantly builds up skin thickness. Please understand that I am not advocating deep peels for most people. Few people have the emotional readiness and the motivation to go through the process. But I want you to know all your options.

A word of caution: If you have telangiectasia and are considering microdermabrasion for some other skin condition, be aware that most microdermabrasion machines suction the skin while abrading, and this vacuuming force may irritate already visible capillaries. Look for a practitioner with a machine that does not have this built-in suctioning element.

THINNING, DRY SKIN

Thin skin comes with time. The natural progression of skin is that eventually, inevitably, the dermis thins, collagen breaks down, and skin becomes more transparent to capillaries and veins, partially due to thinning and partially due to subcutaneous fat loss.

Dryness also comes with time. Even if you started out with normal skin, or perhaps even a bit oily skin, you may join the ranks of the dry-skinned after menopause.

The loss of estrogen after menopause is a major contributor to both the thinness and the dryness of aging skin.

In terms of skin care, it would serve you well to do something that might seem ordinarily counterintuitive: Focus intently on the skin stimulation phase of my skin-care program.

At sixty-seven, Cynthia was beautiful, except for the excessive dryness of her thin, very light skin, with visible capillaries. Because she was afraid of irritation, she'd always used very rich night and day creams.

I explained the benefit of glycolic acid pads to her and prescribed a thin serum for collagen stimulation, rich in carnosine and glycolic, lactic, and salicylic acids, with vitamin E and bioactive amino acid peptides. I also gave her a lipid-based serum to re-create the protective lipid barrier she needed. I calmed her concerns about irritation with assurances that if any irritation developed, it would not be harmful. She could simply stop using the products and it would go away. Otherwise, no pain, no gain.

Three weeks later, she returned with visibly softer lines around the eyes and more even-toned skin. She was delighted. The feeling of dryness in her skin was gone for the first time ever, she told me. She was totally surprised that rich creams had never accomplished what a strong acidic serum in combination with the right skin-identical lipids had.

Thin, dry skin can benefit from superficial, medium, and deep peels as well, whether chemical, mechanical, or laser. If, after a superficial peel, you sustain redness longer than you think you should, do not panic. Light peels cannot cause any lasting damage under any conditions. When you recover, your skin will look better than you expected. And, as you know by now, the deeper the peel, the better the results.

Having grown up in Arizona, fifty-eight-year-old Katherine had severely sun-damaged skin, full of age spots, lines, and red capillaries. She looked her age and then some. Three weeks after undergoing a deep peel, she was still bright red and unable to go back to work. She was very distressed. She felt she'd never been through anything so difficult, and she was worried that she'd never recover.

I just smiled and asked her to look in the mirror. How many years did the procedure take off your face? I asked.

"Well, without the redness, I looked like this about twelve years ago," she replied.

"Wait," I advised.

Three months later, she was still a bit red, but by then she was convinced that the color would soon fade, and she was thoroughly appreciative of the procedure that had turned back the clock on her looks. "It was the best decision I ever made," she told me.

SAGGING AROUND THE JAW
AND LOSS OF NECK ANGULATION

In all honesty, sagging around the jawline is a surgical problem. While deep nasolabial folds or marionette lines at the corner of the mouth can be greatly improved by injecting fillers, the jawline cannot be helped by Botox or any other injected filler substance.

A sagging jawline is the number one indication for a face-lift; nothing else will make it go away.

Unfortunately, many unscrupulous businesspeople will try to tell you differently. For instance, a year ago, I saw a mask available in England that, the promotion claimed, would lift the jawline until you washed the mask off. Essentially, it is a glue that binds the skin together. If you use it, you'll need to make sure not to let anyone get too close, because the glue can be seen on the skin, and it looks exactly like what it is: a mask. The manufacturer will try to tell you that it has a permanent effect by "retraining the muscles." Do not fall for that; it is impossible.

Worse yet, there are people who will try to tell you that a topical serum can visibly and permanently tighten a sagging jawline. They have only one thing in mind: their retirement account.

It is impossible to apply a serum and have it tighten a sagging jawline, and the reason is very simple. The aging process is more than skin-deep. It affects bones, muscles, and ligaments as well as the dermis and subcutaneous fat. So how can anyone claim that there is a magic serum that when applied to the skin will take care of the aging of all these structures underneath? All these potions do is dry your skin. It feels tight because it's dry, so you could be fooled into thinking that the skin is actually tightening around the muscle. It's not—and there's no visible change. Despite what many advertisers would have you believe, there is no face-lift in a bottle.

A sagging jawline happens because of a combination of thinning skin, loss of subcutaneous fat, loss of muscle bulk, and loss of bone in the cheeks and jaw—the same factors that account for jowls. The ninety-degree angle between the neck and the chin is also lost as we age for these same reasons, plus the fact that the muscles and tendons in the neck change consistency and are less able to follow the chinline. This is why Botox injections in the neck can help relax the muscles and temporarily reduce the loss of angulation.

A few decades ago, plastic surgery was only concerned with the skin. Surgeons pulled the skin tight, and that was that. Unfortunately, that is how it looked, too: skin pulled tight over atrophied muscle, shrunken bone, and absent fat. These days, plastic surgery is far more sophisticated. Surgeons address missing fat and tighten loose muscles so the resulting look is a lot more natural.

"You can't perceive good plastic surgery," says my friend Dr. Julian Henley, a master of natural-looking surgery, "whereas you can tell bad plastic surgery a block away."

A deep peel does help the jawline to a small extent because of its remarkable skin-tightening capacity.

You may have heard that facial exercises can tighten the face. Since wrinkles are caused by moving and exercising the face, I can't see how it can work.

As far as topical skin care is concerned: Keep using strong, scientifically based products as your best weapons against skin aging. Help yourself further by engaging in a healthy lifestyle: Don't smoke, and stay out of the sun.

SKIN-CARE FALLACIES

Muscles can be retrained to lift a sagging jawline. Don't believe it if the manufacturer of a mask or cream tries to tell you so. Unfortunately, the only truly effective treatment for a sagging jawline is surgery.

- *Thin, fair, Caucasian skin is fragile and less resilient to laser or acid peels.* Not true. Darker skin tones are more sensitive and vulnerable by far.

- *If you have a dull complexion, you must go to a doctor for a chemical peel or dermabrasion.* Fortunately, the problem of sallow skin can be solved at home with results that are comparable to what can be provided by superficial peels in a doctor's office.

- *If, after a superficial peel, you sustain redness longer than you think you should, it means something has gone wrong.* Not at all. Light peels cannot cause any lasting damage under any conditions. When you recover, your skin will look better than you expected.

CHAPTER SEVEN

YOUR CONSULTATION WITH DR. DENESE

Let us look in the mirror once again and try to diagnose and solve some skin problems together. Of course, I wish I could be there to see your skin and talk to you. I am currently working on a new interactive Web site that will someday allow us to have a two-way encounter, but for now, I can try to explain the major signs of neglect that appear on our faces as we age and what can be done about them.

Of course, "neglect" may not be the right word. Few of us would purposely neglect our faces. We are perhaps more narcissistic about our facial skin than any other part of our body. We all are intensely invested in what it looks like because it reflects our age and personality, and makes us feel attractive and desirable.

Now take an objective look at your face. Please, do not use a magnifying mirror. The world does not see you with a magnifying glass, so why upset yourself for no reason? I doubt there are many people—if any—who could look at their skin that closely, with all the imperfections exaggerated, and be happy with what they see. Personally I have decent skin, but I know I would be troubled by what a magnifying mirror would show me.

LET'S LOOK AT YOUR FOREHEAD

Do you see vertical lines between your eyebrows? These are sometimes referred to as the "number 11" between the brows. Do you have horizontal lines on your forehead?

These wrinkles come about for two reasons: collagen breakdown, primarily as a result of sun exposure, and the muscle pull under the skin. If you have a habit of drawing your eyebrows together or wrinkling your forehead, these lines will happen sooner rather than later, and they will grow deeper and deeper unless you do something.

What can you do?

Since there are two main sources of the wrinkle—the skin and the muscle—ideally, you should treat both.

As far as muscles are concerned, these lines may be significantly helped by Botox injections, if you want to go that route. Try it once and see if it is for you. The results can be impressive.

You can also try serums that contain muscle-relaxing agents for more modest results—or use them in conjunction with Botox to extend the life expectancy of your expensive injections. These days, the most sophisticated skin relaxing products, the active ingredients—Argireline (acetyl hexopeptide-3), collagen, and vitamin antioxidants among them—are delivered in a liposomal system. Liposomes are highly complex, microscopic lipid (fatty) spheres that encapsulate water and other ingredients. Enclosing an ingredient within a liposome entraps it as "payload," keeping it fresh. Liposome encapsulation also improves an ingredient's concentration and duration at the target site.

After addressing the muscles, we need a treatment to build up the skin. We need to exfoliate first, so whatever we put on the skin will penetrate more deeply. Then we need to bring in collagen-building ingredients. AHA/BHA, vitamin C, and retinol are all excellent. However, also greatly effective are the bioactive amino acid peptides, sometimes called oligopeptides (oligo means few). These are short-chain amino acid peptides, small enough to penetrate the skin. They can directly stimulate the cellular machinery called fibroblasts, involved in making skin collagen. Fibroblast cells are your skin's best friends because they are the primary manufacturers of collagen and elastin, which assures skin elasticity. We have many fibroblasts in the skin when we are young, and—you guessed it—we lose them as we grow older, so our collagen supply becomes less than perfect. These powerful oligopeptides can change the course of your skin's history to some extent and, as the pharmaceutical companies continue to perfect them, they hold the promise of bringing previously unimaginable results to wrinkle reduction. One of the early peptides, trademarked as Matrixyl, can be found in a product named StriVectin-SD. D–StriVectin was originally made for the body, therefore when you use it on your face it can prove to be too oily. StriVectin-SD is a good beginning, but soon there will be newer and more effective peptides in the marketplace.

The way in which peptides are prepared for delivery in a product is key. They are fragile, and to survive in a cream or serum, they need to be coated for protection. Encapsulation keeps them fresh until they reach your skin and enables them to penetrate more effectively into the lower layers of the skin.

Another ingredient on the cutting edge of biotechnology is epidermal growth factor (EPF), a healing agent derived from recombinant DNA/RNA that directly stimulates collagen production. It has received much publicity recently and is present in a few skin-care products. The problem with it at the moment is the price. One gram of EPF (about the size of a pinch of salt) can cost as much as $250,000! How much of this substance can you put into a jar of cream? Until the price comes down, I think products containing bioactive oligopeptides are a more viable alternative. As with all skin care, percentage is key. We have developed an oligopeptide product with three times the oligopeptides of the industy standard (Triple-strength Wrinkle Smoother).

LET'S LOOK AT THE FINE LINES AROUND YOUR EYES

Do you see lines around the eyes when you are *not* smiling—or only when you are? This is an important distinction, because a different treatment is required depending on how you answer.

If you have lines around your eyes *only* when you are smiling, then the lines are of muscular origin and have to be treated accordingly. Botox injections can help significantly. You may also consider using topical skin-relaxing alternatives in addition to the injection to extend its life or instead, if you have an aversion to needles (see pages 90–91).

If you have lines around your eyes even when you are not smiling, then you need to step up your skin collagen-building effort in addition to treating the muscle component. If the lines around your eyes are deep, there comes a point when Botox injections become counterproductive. If you have heavy lines around your eyes, Boxtox can actually prompt lines to gather under the eyes and appear to be more plentiful, at least for the duration of the injection's effectiveness. An ethical doctor can advise you if Botox would help or hurt in your case.

One of the greatest challenges in skin care is to build collagen around the delicate area of the eyes. The traditional collagen builders, such as glycolic acid and retinol, are much too irritating for the eye area in any meaningful concentrations. Oligopeptides are highly effective; less irritating; and, in my opinion, the best substances for building collagen around the eye area. The encapsulated versions in a light serum are preferable for better preservation, delivery, and penetration. Some good products to try are StriVectin-SD Eye Cream Reviva Labs Peptides and More Anti-Wrinkle Cream, Cellular Skin Rx Eye Bright

Treatment Serum, Dermalogica Intensive Eye Repair, and my own RestorEyes.

Protecting the eye area from sun damage is more important than for any other part of the face. SPF 30 protection should be applied in all seasons, rain or shine.

Dryness is a critical issue around the eye area because this part of the face has the fewest oil glands. Even if your skin is oily, the eye region may be dry. And if your skin is dry, your eye area is likely to be very uncomfortable without substantial lipid replacement. The lipids should be *skin-identical* as much as possible. Ceramides and essential fatty acids are the best choices. Do not be misled by terms such as "natural plant oils." Natural plant oils are great for a plant's skin, but not for yours. Your best choice is a lipid closest to your own natural skin lipids. The right lipids may be able to repair the all-important protective skin lipid barrier and to prevent water loss and subsequent drying of the delicate eye area. A good eye cream should feel rich and moisturizing, although oftentimes it might look oily and shiny for the entire day. Until recently, consumers had to make a difficult choice: to maintain a good, matte look around the eye area at the expense of feeling dry all day; or to look shiny, but feel comfortable in this area. In my opinion, no one has to make such a choice any longer. These days there are a few eye creams that feel rich yet won't leave you looking shiny. Dermalogica makes one called Intensive Eye Repair. RestorEyes, by Denese products, is uniquely rich in Ceramides, Retinol, and essential fatty acids. It feels rich beyond compare, yet has no shine at all. It can hold moisture the entire day, yet no one has to see it.

LET'S LOOK AT THE AREA UNDER YOUR EYES

Do you have prominent under-eye circles? Do you need to use an under-eye concealer much of the time?

There is a simple diagnostic method I would like to teach you before you spend hundreds of dollars on expensive eye care that is based on a false premise.

Under-eye circles are a special condition. If you have them and you do *not* have severe wrinkles under your eyes, we have some work we can do.

Let me tell you about a patient of mine, Katrina, a pretty forty-two-year-old brunette who came to see me because of ever-increasing dark circles under her eyes. She told me that she'd always had a slight fullness under her eyes, even as a youngster, but now the circles were starting to qualify as bags. She said that for the past ten years, she'd spent hundreds of dollars on gels and creams that promised to "drain" the fluid from under her eyes and reduce the puffiness—all to no avail.

I was not surprised. There is no topical product that will "drain puffiness" from under the eyes. Although there are many products, some very high-end ones, making such claims on the basis of some herbal or other ingredient, to the best of my knowledge, science has not progressed so far. Katrina felt that her problem was getting worse with each passing year and, to her dismay, she believed she was starting to look exactly like her mother, with prominent under-eye protrusions.

She did not have many lines under the eyes. In fact, her skin was quite taut. But she did have noticeable under-eye circles. While we looked in a mirror together, I took a Q-tip, pushed on one of the bags, and watched the darkness disappear. This showed us that the darkness of the circle was not inherent to the skin. It was merely a shadow cast by the eye bag. The bag itself was very small, and Katrina was really more troubled by the shadow.

How do bags develop under the eyes, and how can you get rid of them? Katrina had a fat pad under each eye that was making her under-eye bags more and more protuberant as the skin became more loose and lax. The fat pad remained the same, but the skin's ability to hold it in was declining with each passing year, so the subsequent shadow was ever-increasing. The best way to solve her problem was to surgically remove the solid fat pad. After this was done, her skin quickly shrank back to normal, and the circle disappeared without a trace. Her recovery was quick—only four days—and she was delighted with the outcome.

If you are troubled by under-eye circles, look at your eye area and answer the following question: Do you have deep wrinkles under the eyes? If not, if the skin is relatively tight, then the problem is not inherent to the skin. Look deeper. You may not realize that there is a fat pad protruding from under your eyes, casting a shadow and creating the circle. Take a Q-tip and push on the under-eye area. If the circle disappears, it indicates a hidden fat pad, and it also indicates that the source of the problem is not the skin. Roll your eyes upward and look as high up in the mirror as you can. Do you see the outline of a fat pad? You may or may not have noticed before that it is there. The only way to get rid of the fat pad is by removing it surgically. You cannot "drain the under-eye puffiness" or "break down the fat," as some of the most outrageous claims on cream jars would like you to believe. Save your money and do not allow anyone to insult your intelligence this way. Look at your relatives. If you see bags under their eyes, chances are bags will be coming your way, too. They do not improve with time. They only get worse. The surgery to correct this problem is an easy procedure, and the results are usually excellent. Be sure to go to an experienced plastic surgeon; you do not want an inexperienced surgeon taking out too much fat from under your eyes.

Circles under the eyes that are an overall dark color and *not* caused by the shadow cast by fat pads are often inherited by people of darker-skinned ethnicities, such as Italian, Indian, African-American, Greek, Portuguese, and Latino. In these cases, the entire under-eye area is dark, not just a circle. This is also an inherited feature that usually grows worse with age—and it's a much more difficult problem to solve. There is no easy solution to it. The condition develops due to the fragility of blood vessels, thinning skin that becomes more and more transparent over time, deposits of dark pigment cells from chronic inflammation, and a lack of fat under the skin to make it less transparent. Vitamin K may help the permeability of the vessels, although the effect will probably be very modest at best. Building up the thickness of the skin could help to lessen the transparency. But a fading cream that breaks down dark pigment discoloration is usually the most helpful. Make sure the fading cream is nonirritating; otherwise it can make the problem worse.

When thirty-seven-year-old Jennifer, who is of Greek descent, came to see me, she was troubled by dark under-eye circles. I saw at once that there was no evidence of fat pads in her case. In fact, she had a hollowed-out look in her under-eye area, which was devoid of any fat padding. We achieved some reasonably good results with carefully dosed botanical fading agents, and I introduced her to an under-eye concealer with built-in botanical skin faders that worked well for her. Unlike the problem fat pads, which can have a good solution, this is a harder problem to solve.

LET'S LOOK AT YOUR NOSE, CHEEKS, AND FOREHEAD

Do you see prominent pores, especially on the cheeks? Clogged pores? Blackheads? Whiteheads? Is there redness? Is the redness from broken capillaries? Or is it more from inflammation as a result of clogged pores?

Assess your condition carefully, because if your diagnosis is correct, you may be able to remedy the situation. If you answered yes to any of the questions above, I can share a few facts to help you avoid making mistakes in how you should treat your skin. But let us start with a case study.

At thirty-six, Daria, a dark-eyed, black-haired beauty, came to see me with problems that can be typical for a woman of Italian descent: porous skin, prominent pores, blackheads, and some redness around the nose in a butterfly distribution, due to clogged pores. She told me that her skin had always been dry, and it felt especially tight after she washed her face. She was convinced that she had very delicate, sensitive skin, which she'd been treating very protectively with creams ever since she was a teenager.

How had she been applying the creams? I wanted to know.

She was very surprised by how I could even ask such a question. "How else?" she said. "I apply it as if I am painting a house, of course. I cover every inch so I don't miss any part of my face."

That was her first mistake.

The nose and the surrounding area that fans out across the cheeks like a butterfly is richly endowed with oil glands, even for someone with dry skin overall. I have yet to see a face with dry skin that ever needed extra oil on the nose. Skin is thicker and oilier on the nose than on any other area of the face, including around the eyes, on the cheeks, and the neck. You cannot treat these areas the same. In fact, I tell all my patients not to put any creams or oily substances on their nose and the surrounding cheeks. Oils are the last things this area needs. If you put more oil on an oily region, all you do is clog pores, increase pore size, and create low-grade inflammation in the area that gives rise to redness. Your own experience may have already taught you this, but it never hurts to clarify. Treat the nose area using all of the steps in my program; clean it with strong glycolic acids; exfoliate; microdermabrade; peel the area; and use thin, water-based serums for anti-aging effect, but do *not* feed this area with lipids. It does not need it. It may only backfire.

DO YOU HAVE REDNESS ON YOUR NOSE, CHEEKS, OR CHIN?

Look in the mirror. Do you see the outline of blood vessels under the skin? Are they red or bluish? If you press on them, do they lose color? Take a Q-tip and press one end of a vessel. Does it lose color? Now press on the other end. Does it lose color now? Whether it blanches or not, tells you the direction of blood flow in the vessel. Doctors do this test before eliminating a vessel with an electrical needle. In general, these surface capillaries are nonfunctional, so they can be taken out without compromising the blood supply to the skin. There are two main ways to eliminate capillaries: electrical desiccation or laser. Of the two, the laser is a bit more reliable. However, capillaries may resurface because if, for some reason, the hemodynamics are such that the blood needs to flow that way, no matter how a vessel is removed, there are no guarantees it won't return.

The key to this diagnostic exercise is to establish exactly what is responsible for the redness. Do you see visible, formed vessels? Or, perhaps, are you seeing redness that is from inflammation caused by clogged pores? This is an important distinction, because the treatment for each condition is different. Treating the source of the inflammation should precede treating the redness, whether it is from clogged pores, lack of exfoliation, overmoisturizing with pore-clogging oils, or skin care that is too harsh (a rare occurrence).

The following case descriptions will help illustrate my point.

Excessive ruddiness around the nose and cheeks was the problem facing Glenda, a fifty-four-year-old, very fair Englishwoman, who told me that the condition had become significantly worse since the onset of her menopause. She had received a lot of sun exposure in earlier years. Like many blue-eyed blondes of her generation, she had loved the way she looked with a tan. But her very white skin had not tolerated it well. As I looked at her, I could see clearly formed multiple red capillaries under the surface of her thin, frail skin. She responded really well to a few laser treatments. Now she returns to see me once or twice a year for maintenance visits.

With her red hair and pale, freckled skin, thirty-four-year-old Moira's Irish heritage was instantly obvious when she came to see me complaining of ruddiness around her nose and cheeks. Her skin was oily, especially around the area of redness, with many clogged pores. It was difficult to discern formed vessels under the skin. The redness was more amorphous, having to do with inflammation secondary to clogged pores and oiliness.

In her case, laser treatment would have helped significantly, but only temporarily. Since it made no sense to treat the skin symptomatically, without trying to address the cause of the symptoms, I put her on an exfoliation-based skin-care regime to address an acne condition. I also gave her a few light chemical peels over the following four weeks and instructed her not to use any creams on the area throughout that time. The problem resolved successfully, without laser treatment.

DO YOU HAVE DARK SKIN DISCOLORATION?

In my practice, another concern that arises frequently is dark skin discoloration: freckles, sun spots, and age spots. It is a source of anguish because, as the ominous-sounding name suggests, age spots give an aged look to the face.

Age spots have to do with sun exposure, almost exclusively. A few notable exceptions include dark spots that develop after deep inflammatory acne; a long-lasting skin rash that turns dark after the inflammation has resolved; and melasma, a hormonally based, deep-skin discoloration.

The only time you may need your magnifying mirror is when you examine your dark spots. In general, only a doctor can positively decide what a dark spot may signify. However, I can give you a few preliminary pointers so you can sleep better before visiting your doctor if you see something suspicious on your face.

First, establish if the dark spot is completely flat or if it has a thickness and dimension to it. In other words, is it only a spot of color, or does it have color plus some additional tissue that would make it a mole? This is important because a simple skin discoloration is treated very differently than a mole, a discolored spot with extra tissue proliferation. Extra tissue growth can be benign; in fact, it most often is, but it still needs to be treated by a doctor.

It is important to keep moles under close review, to recognize the warning signs of melanoma or other forms of skin cancer. There are four signs to watch for, the ABCDs of melanoma:

- Asymmetry: if one half of the mole does not match the other

- Border: any irregular border in a mole is significant

- Color: variegated color is a warning sign (multicolored: light, dark, darker, red, etc.)

- Diameter: if it is larger than 5 mm (about the size of the head of a pencil eraser)

Also, if a mole begins to itch or starts to change suddenly, you have no time to waste. You must see a doctor. Melanoma occurs mostly in areas that have been sun-exposed—however, sometimes it can surface in regions of lesser sun exposure as well. On the other hand, basal cell carcinoma is strongly related to sun exposure.

I'll never forget a patient I encountered while I was a medical student at Sloan Kettering Memorial Hospital at Cornell University Medical College. David was a vibrant young man of forty-six, an executive, husband, father, and former Marine who'd had a lot of unprotected sun exposure while he was in the service. Later he became an avid golfer and spent many more hours in the sun. When he developed a dark spot on his left ear, it was small, but had an irregular border, uneven color, and lacked symmetry. The diagnosis of a malignant melanoma was made promptly, but still, it was too late. His cancer had spread, and he was gone in only eight months.

Melanoma is one of the most vicious forms of cancer, and once you see a case, you never face the sun the same way again. I hope I can convey the importance of constant and consistent sun protection.

Back to something less sad: cosmetic skin care. Look at your age spots under a 3X mirror. Inspect the spot that bothers you. If it is completely flat, traditional skin-fading methods may have a chance of working. However, if the age spot is raised even a tiny bit, if you see any extra tissue over it, traditional skin-fading methods will fail, so do not waste any time on them. Show the spot to a doctor and ask his or her advice.

Skin discolorations are difficult to treat. Over-the-counter products rarely succeed. Even doctor-prescribed products (usually a combination of hydroquinone, glycolic acid, and Retin A) often have disappointing results. Light or superficial chemical peels and light microdermabrasion are often advertised as a solution to age spots, but I strongly disagree. Do not spend money on these procedures in the hopes of getting rid of age spots, because you may be disappointed. However, medium-depth laser or chemical peels have a high success rate; remember, they require at least a week's recovery time. Anything less will simply be inadequate to address the problem.

LET'S LOOK AT YOUR OVERALL FACE: DRY, OILY, AND COMBINATION SKIN

DO YOU HAVE DRY SKIN?

Are you near or over fifty? Do you have dry lines on your face? Do you think your skin is dry?

These are fascinating questions. The following case study will illustrate why.

Geri, a spirited, fifty-seven-year-old redhead, was so focused on her career, she didn't worry much about her skin, other than being convinced that it was dry. She was freckled and had had her share of the sun in her youth, when she hadn't known any better. She had dry lines all over her face, especially in areas of intense muscle movement; overall, there was a coarse, rough, and dry quality to her skin. She treated it with rich, very expensive moisturizing creams twice a day, but no serums and no meaningful exfoliation. She also had some clogged pores on her forehead and around her nose, probably as a consequence of the rich and clogging creams she was using.

My assessment of her skin was that it wasn't really dry at all. The dryness she felt most likely had to do with a significant buildup of old dead cells on the skin surface that appeared as dry, rough skin. I put her on a strict exfoliation program of daily glycolic peel pads; microdermabrasion cream twice a week; and thin, acid-based serums rich in amino acid peptides for collagen stimulation. She used a thicker serum as her last step to seal the skin at night and during the day, but no creams. Three weeks later, her skin looked remarkably different. Her friends and acquaintances started asking her what she was doing with her skin. They wanted to know her secret. Her dry lines were dramatically improved, and the rough, dry quality of her skin disappeared. She no longer felt that her skin was dry, even though she was no longer using her creams. By exfoliating and using the right lipids, moisture was finally reaching her skin, and that proved to be the solution to her "dry skin" problem.

If you feel that dry skin is your most serious problem, start an aggressive exfoliation and collagen stimulation program, even though it is counterintuitive, and see how your skin responds.

Be sure to use the right lipids, the skin-identical kind. You can know you are using the right lipids on your skin if the serum or cream penetrates and disappears into your skin within a few minutes. If it lingers on the skin surface as a shiny residue for hours, it is not absorbing into your skin properly. It is the wrong product for you, so get rid of it. It is merely sitting on top, sealing from the outside, possibly even clogging pores. The right moisturizer supports the skin lipid barrier from the inside of the *stratum corneum* (the upper layer of the epidermus), so it is not visible as a shiny layer on the outside. It disappears into the skin within a few minutes and provides internal support.

Few of us start out in life with dry skin, but nearly all of us will end up there after menopause.

A woman in her twenties with thin, dry skin presents the picture of perfection. The skin is clogged-pore-free and line-free, an even-colored ideal that everyone dreams about. Unfortunately, thin, dry skin, especially if it is fair and exposed to the sun, ages fast—the fastest.

Eva, a nineteen-year-old model from the Czech Republic who barely spoke English, was a tall, natural blonde with the kind of flawless, lineless skin that most of us can only dream of. She came into my office to buy cream because her face "felt dry." She told me that she'd never tanned in her life. She wanted a cream with sunscreen that she could use every day. I thought I hadn't heard her right. Normally, with other young women her age, I have the tedious job of trying to convince them of the importance of sun protection, and I often run into a lot of resistance. I suppose, when you come to this country hoping to make a living with your face, you grow up fast.

Most dry skins are thin and show signs of aging rapidly. By the time a woman with dry skin is in her mid-thirties, there are usually lines around her eyes, especially if she's had a history of sun exposure. Her skin will look and feel dry, particularly around the eyes, where sebaceous glands are the least prevalent. This trend will continue into her forties and fifties, with the skin growing thinner and becoming progressively drier. After menopause there is a dramatic loss in skin thickness, with even further increases in dryness that never improve. So even if you start out with normal to oily skin, eventually you may end up with dry and thin skin as time goes by.

The objective of treatment for dry skin is fourfold:

1. Anti-aging skin care, which involves stimulating the skin's own collagen-building machinery with strong ingredients such as glycolic acids, AHA/BHA, retinol, bioactive oligopeptides, vitamin C, and/or prescription-strength tretinoins (Renova, Retin A). Many of these ingredients may be so irritating to thin, dry skin that it is a true challenge to find a happy medium.

2. Halting collagen breakdown from sun exposure by adopting the habit of using SPF 30 every day of the year.

3. Re-creating the skin lipid barrier, if necessary several times a day, to protect the skin from water loss.

4. Exfoliating. One of the main reasons why skin can feel dry is because of a thick, dead layer of cells on the surface that does not allow proper moisture penetration.

When a woman has dry skin, she often tends to be very protective of it and focuses nearly all of her skin-care efforts on re-creating the skin lipid barrier or the "feel good" stage of skin maintenance. She washes with a mild cleanser, then puts on a cream for the night and another cream in the morning. Maybe, if she's lucky, the day cream has an SPF 15 in it, but that's about all.

Of course, I can't cast any blame. The entire skin-care establishment has been focused on the single objective of the "feel good" stage of re-creating the skin lipid barrier since time immemorial, because this is what sells best. If it has served you properly, good for you. But if you have been disappointed by "feel good" creams in the past, it is time to try something new. Try my six-step program. Use the glycolic pads only two days a week and gradually increase as your tolerance grows. Use a microdermabrasion cream once a week.

If the acid-based serum causes you to develop any irritation, don't panic. This simply means that you are overusing the product, so just cut back on the application. You have done no harm to your skin. Wait until the irritation goes away, then gradually resume application until you find your own pace. You may consider serums with some muscle-relaxing properties as a preventive measure as well, or try a Botox injection for the same reasons.

Next comes the skin lipid barrier phase. Make sure that the serum or cream you are using contains ceramides and essential fatty acids that are skin-identical lipids for human skin. Coconut oil or avocado oil is great for the skin of the avocado or the coconut, but not for yours.

Please review chapter 5, "Winning the Wrinkle War," for even more techniques to prevent and improve facial lines. Thin, dry skin can benefit remarkably from more invasive skin-rejuvenating procedures.

DO YOU HAVE OILY, ACNE-PRONE SKIN?

There is a saying that "oily skin is a blessing in disguise." Interestingly enough, people with oily skin are the last to agree. I rarely see patients as desperate, as ready for treatment, as those suffering from oily skin. True, oily skin wrinkles less in midlife and beyond, but there lies a long and rocky road before you get there.

Let's look at one extreme case of oiliness and discover what we can learn from the remarkable success I had with this patient.

Esther was a fifty-four-year-old nurse with extremely oily skin. She no longer had acne breakouts, but her many craterlike acne scars told a story about her struggles with deep cystic acne, even up to just a few years earlier. She could not wear makeup or powder; it came off within an hour, and her face was perpetually shiny. She washed her face several times a day but even then she never felt that she was presentable.

She did not have a single line on her face, but, sadly, she had the worst case of oiliness I had seen in all the years of my practice. I gave her a 30 percent salicylic acid peel, which is a light, BHA chemical peel intended to dissolve oily plugs in pores, break down oil in general, and exfoliate the top layer of the skin.

She called me three days later to say that her skin had never looked better. Now she could go through a day without washing her face. She was able to put on powder and not look very shiny. "Can I come back for another peel?" she asked. "I need one again."

Normally I would give a peel of this depth only once every two weeks, at best, but I told her to come in and let me see what we could do. Five days later, I did give her another peel—and with great success.

Three days after that, she called again, respectfully demanding yet another peel. She lived two hours away by car, so eventually I taught her how to do the peels for herself; she was a nurse, after all. She also started to do home microdermabrasion, with an abrasive cream, daily. She is delighted with the outcome because now her oiliness problem is under complete control and she has great, thick skin with very few lines.

Esther's was clearly an extreme case of oiliness. But what worked for her tells us what works for oily skin in general.

When you have oily skin, your main objectives are threefold:

1. Dissolve the sebaceous oil product promptly so it does not have a chance to clog the pores and follicles; give rise to blackheads, whiteheads, acne, or enlarged pores; or cause a generally reddish, inflammatory skin condition.

2. Exfoliate—remove dead surface skin cells so as not to promote pore clogging.

3. Use anti-aging skin care.

Many of my patients with oily skin feel left out when it comes to anti-aging skin care because they cannot put creams on their face. The good news is that objective number three is taken care of automatically by the agents that are used to achieve goals one and two.

Exfoliating with glycolic acid or AHA-based acids is the first key step.

I think that a glycolic acid or AHA/BHA–based cleansing pad is the best solution to bring AHA/BHA into the skin. An AHA/BHA cleanser or toner could not possibly qualify as sufficient exfoliation and sebaceous gland treatment. Please, do not let anyone convince you to the contrary. And *an exfoliating cream containing glycolic acid is also not a good idea for oily skin.* Why keep the sebaceous product on the skin overnight? A pad that you wipe your face with and throw away makes the most sense to me. You should use the pads at least once, but more likely twice a day, as long as you can tolerate them well.

The pad should create a tingle on your skin; otherwise you are not getting what you need out of it. It's difficult to find a pad with enough active ingredients in a broad, commercial brand. Broad-distribution commercial brands are designed to cause no complaints from any segment of the population, from a twenty-two-year-old man with an oily complexion, to a seventy-eight-year-old woman with dry, thin skin. How could any product satisfy all these different skin types except by making the product so weak that it may achieve nothing at the end? You are better off looking for an AHA/glycolic acid pad in some of the doctor-brand products.

If the pad is advertised as a salicylic acid pad (BHA only), beware. Although salicylic acid is excellent to achieve the goals of oily skin care, manufacturers are only allowed by law to put a maximum of 2 percent of salicylic acid in the products, which is not useful for your purposes. Do not buy a BHA pad unless it is a combination of AHA/BHA so you'll get the tingle you need. Use a home microdermabrasion cream as well, several times a week.

If you have oily skin, you can also use some of the advanced, acid-based, thin serums that are rich in skin-stimulating ingredients and antioxidants, such as bioactive oligopeptides, vitamin C, carnosine, CoQ10, alphalipoic acid, and others. These valuable ingredients are always best delivered in an acidic medium because the acidic base helps skin permeation. If you have oily or combination skin you are in luck, because you will have no trouble tolerating these serums.

Prescription-strength tretinoic acid (Retin A, Differin) also serves a dual purpose by regulating the sebaceous glands and by acting as a powerful anti-aging agent for your skin. Realize that prescription-strength, tretinoin-based products can dry the skin significantly, especially around the eyes and the corners of the mouth. One of my patients once called me in a panic after using Retin A on her face for four days. She was seeing more lines around her eyes than she had before. It *can* be a frightening experience to use these medications if you do not realize that the dry lines they induce are temporary. It may take a while for them to resolve, but nevertheless, they are temporary. The lines to fear, the permanent ones, develop slowly and insidiously, not overnight.

Even if you have oily skin, your eye area still needs to be treated as dry skin. There might be an exception to this rule, but I have yet to see it. It may be counterintuitive to you if you're used to trying to control oil on your skin, but you need to keep the eye area well supplied with skin-identical lipids.

If you have oily skin, I do not recommend putting creams on your face, especially on the oiliest regions—the nose, the chin, and the forehead. Your thin serums will take care of the anti-aging issues in these areas. Creams are likely to get you into trouble with clogged pores, and there is no need for their barrier function in these areas.

Oily skin also responds well to superficial chemical peels and microdermabrasion, but it does *not* respond well to traditional cleaning facials. The traditional idea of cleaning the skin pore by pore can cause more redness, breakouts, and irritation, especially in light of the fact that traditional facials were designed for dry, more mature skin, so all the cleansers, serums, and creams that are part of the traditional facial protocol are not meant for your oily skin. Chemical peels and microdermabrasion, on the other hand, address all the pores at the same time and open those that are ready to be opened. These procedures need to be repeated a few times for best results.

DO YOU HAVE COMBINATION SKIN?

Most of us have normal to combination skin, which turns progressively drier and thinner after menopause.

In my opinion, there is no such thing as a uniformly oily, dry, or normal skin. Oily skin can be dry around the eyes, and dry skin can be oily on the nose and forehead. So normal-to-combination skin has to be treated as dry skin around the eyes and maybe the cheek area, and as oily skin on the nose, chin, and part of the forehead (the T-zone), at least in most cases.

The skin-care establishment has creams for normal-to-combination skin, although I question how a "one size fits all cream" can be useful. The "normal" cream may be too dry for the eye area and too oily for the nose and forehead. I realize it may be inconvenient to give each skin area what it needs, but I believe it is better to do so than under-moisturize the eye area while overmoisturizing the nose and forehead and possibly creating clogged pores.

There are only a few general principles we have to keep in mind to give each area what it needs. By now, you probably know these principles already.

We need to exfoliate all over, but definitely more so in the oily areas of the T-zone, so we need to spend more time here with the glycolic pad and the microdermabrasion cream.

All parts of the skin need skin stimulation from thin, highly pene-trating serums rich in bioactive peptides, vitamins, carnosine, AHA/BHA, antioxidants, etc. However, you have to be light-handed with the serum in the eye area because it may dry and irritate. Apply it less often there, at least until you are used to it.

However, not all parts of the skin need the phase that re-creates the lipid barrier. The oil-rich T-zone, or perhaps just the nose, does not need the lipid barrier serum. So be heavy-handed with the serum in the eye area, but give little or none to the areas that are already heavy in oil production.

The same applies to the final sealant: the night cream. Use it richly where it is needed, and skip skin areas where you are oily. Applying a cream is not like painting a room; it is more like painting a canvas. Put the cream where you need it and do not put it where you don't. Trust your instincts; you know best. Remember: the primary purpose of a cream is to function as a barrier. Oily areas do not need barriers; they have their own.

FINALLY, LET'S LOOK AT SKIN COLOR

If you have dark skin, you can be thankful because:

- You will wrinkle less as a result of the inherent sun protection you receive from skin pigment (unless, of course, you are reckless in the sun).

- Darker skins tend to be thicker, another reason why you will wrinkle less and age better, in general.

Now let's look at the downside.

Darker skins are more sensitive to potentially irritating ingredients such as prescription-strength tretinoins (Retin A, Renova) and high-percentage AHA/BHA acids. If you overirritate dark skin, it will hyperpigment (turn darker) in places of irritation. In most cases the darkening is temporary; however, you still have to be careful. This means you have to be cautious with the skin-building phase and avoid potential irritation. On the other hand, darker skin needs less skin-building as a result of inherently thicker skin and less sun-related collagen damage.

Dark skin is less tolerant of professional resurfacing procedures. For instance, a doctor has to be much more careful in performing an acid peel or aggressive microdermabrasion on dark skin because the patient may develop temporary (or possibly permanent) hyperpigmentation. In fact, the deepest peel that can be performed on a dark skin is a medium-depth peel that is best suited to remove hyperpigmentary changes.

The most important aging issue for dark skin is hyperpigmentary changes. For darker skins, this is the most important factor that distinguishes a young face from an older one. Dark skin becomes darker in certain parts over the years. Around the mouth area—an area of a lot of movement—the skin becomes invariably darker. The forehead becomes darker, sometimes not evenly, but in blotches. The eye area stays relatively light. The cheeks become darker in blotches, especially if the person suffered from acne. The dark, postacne marks can be visible on the cheeks or forehead for years (sometimes many years, depending on the severity of the acne).

My patient, Mary, a dignified, sixty-seven-year-old Jamaican lady, was a registered nurse, trained in England. She took great pride in her work with the terminally ill. She came to me asking for help to make her face even-colored, as it used to be.

"I would like the same color all over my face as I have around my eye and cheek areas," she said. She had no lines to speak of and, as she correctly saw it, the only "older" features on her face were the darker regions around her mouth and large dark blotches on her forehead. "If I could be as light as I am around my eyes, I would look a lot younger," she said, and I agreed with her completely.

Evening out skin tone in dark skin is a difficult balancing act. The accumulated melanocytes, which are responsible for darkness, are deeply seated in the skin and cannot be conveniently removed by microdermabrasion or light acid peels. I often get annoyed when I see home-care microdermabrasion creams marketed to dark skins as something that "with sufficient scrubbing, can lighten and even out skin color." If only it were that easy. The more the poor patient scrubs, the more likely the skin will turn darker in a few days.

Professional microdermabrasion has to be delicately applied as well. Please, do not fall for claims that after a few sessions of in-office microdermabrasion procedures the skin will turn lighter and more even in color. Large sums of money are spent based on these false promises every year simply because the harder the technician uses the mircodermabrasion machine on dark skins, the more likely the skin will turn darker as a result of irritation. It seems like a no-win situation and it really is, if we attempt to remove dark discoloration and even out color by mechanical means only. We need some chemistry here.

There is an agent called hydroquinone, which can inhibit the formation of melanocyte cells that are responsible for dark pigmentary changes. There are also a few other botanical agents that serve similar functions with less irritation, but right now the only FDA-approved skin-fading agent in the United States is hydroquinone. Hydroquinone in over-the-counter strength, which is 2 percent, is not useful, so do not count on it. Hydroquinone by itself, even at the prescription strength of 4 percent, is also not very useful. There are prescription creams that combine hydroquinone with glycolic acid as a penetration facilitator, but in my experience, patients are more often disappointed than not.

The best facilitator for hydroquinone seems to be prescription-strength Retin A, as it is combined in the Obagi NuDerm skin-fading system, which has become the gold standard for evening out the color of dark skins. Retin A is irritating for dark skin; however, the parallel administration of hydroquinone continues to inhibit dark cell formation, and the end result of the combination is a remarkable skin-fading and skin-evening effect. If applied correctly, it rarely fails. Patients often ask me if there is any danger that they will wind up looking like Michael Jackson. No, I tell them, it is impossible. To look like him, you would have to go through highly invasive skin peeling procedures with weeks of recovery that most ethical doctors would not be willing to perform.

In Mary's case, I started her on a combination of Retin A and hydroquinone. After a few weeks of significant redness, peeling, dryness, and irritation, she became uniform in color all over the face and, as she had suspected, she looked years younger. The process is not easy. It can even be frightening at times for laypeople. I think her training as a nurse helped her go through it.

One of the most important things you can do if you have dark skin is avoid the sun; use significant sun block every day of the year; and avoid acne outbreaks as much as possible, because the dark aftermath of acne outbreaks is very long-lasting in dark skin. Seek a doctor's help for acne as soon as possible.

What can you do if discoloration is your problem, but you are not yet prepared to go the harsh way? Exfoliation is key to preventing oily clogs and chronic, low-grade skin inflammation that can darken the skin. The glycolic pads and home microdermabrasion creams can be very useful, too, as long as you realize that you are using them for prevention rather than for a fading effect. Light, acid-based, skin-building serums can be useful as well. Beware of heavy barrier function creams, however. Use them around the eyes or other dry areas, but be careful not to clog the skin.

DO YOU HAVE LIGHT SKIN WITH DARK DISCOLORATIONS?

If you have light skin with many sun spots and age spots, one of the first things to do is to realize that even if you are not "sitting out in the sun," you are still getting too much sun or you have gotten too much sun at some point in the past when you did not know any better.

If you have many dark spots, you have significant sun damage, which means that you need significant, scientifically based skin care. You are not a candidate for just "feel good," traditional skin care, even if you feel that you have sensitive skin and are concerned that you may damage your skin.

When Bethany, a beautiful, forty-six-year-old natural blonde who loves outdoor sports, realized all the damage the sun was causing to her skin, it was much too late. She grew up on the beach and had been working on maintaining a great tan ever since she was a young child. She was very intelligent, so she realized that her worse than average skin damage was going to require more than average effort to reverse. She was quick to let go of her old ideas of using a cream-based system with hardly any exfoliation and eager to try new methods contrary to traditional skin-care protocol. Even though she initially thought her skin was frail, she started aggressive exfoliation (gradually, so as to not get irritated), using several acid-based, ingredient-rich skin-building serums and barrier function skin serums and creams. She also had a medium-depth peel that removed many of her discolorations, and she continued to be a connoisseur of scientifically advanced skin care, with a great sense of adventure. Compared to her sun-worshiping contemporaries, her skin looked like time was standing still for her, even going backward a bit.

Science cannot make you look twenty again, but like Bethany, it can make you look like you have not aged in the past few years. And when you look at the faces of your less open-minded and less adventurous friends, this is saying a lot.

CHAPTER EIGHT

TAMING ACNE

Acne (also known as the bane of our existence) is a chronic inflammatory disease of the sebaceous hair follicles.

How does acne begin? Acne is associated with some swelling, redness, a pustular lesion (pimple) that is followed by a red mark that may turn dark and in some instances may leave a permanent, pitted scar.

Each hair follicle contains a tiny hair and many sebaceous glands. Normally, the sebum, which is the oily substance made by the sebaceous glands, travels up the hair follicle and out to the skin's surface. If for some reason the pores are clogged by old dead skin cells, debris, and overproduction of sebum, you guessed it, the sebum *does not travel* outside. It gets trapped within the follicle.

Normally the skin surface is loaded with bacteria, but the bacteria just sit on the skin and do not cause much trouble. However, when the pore is clogged with sebum, the bacteria happily settle in the clogged pores and you wake up in the morning, see a pimple, and say, *"Oh, no, not another one!"* (The name of the bacteria involved is *Propionobacterium acnes* [*P. acnes*], just in case you want to know who to say "thank you" to.)

The main categories of acne are:

1. Blackheads and whiteheads, also known as open versus closed comedones. These are not, strictly speaking, acne, because there is no inflammation and therefore no redness associated with them.

2. Ordinary acne (also known as inflammatory pustules) is what you would normally call pimples. These pustules include bacterial infection and inflammation, and redness of sebaceous glands.

3. Deep red nodular acne (also known as cystic acne)—inflamed, red, pustular acne with a deep nodular base. This is the most serious form of acne.

4. Rosacea is not actually acne but a related condition, so we'll deal with it later in this chapter.

BLACKHEADS, WHITEHEADS, AND WHAT TO DO ABOUT THEM

Both blackheads and whiteheads are caused by clogged pores, most often a consequence of excess sebaceous production and lack of exfoliation.

Blackheads are *open comedones*—you can see the horrible content of a mix of sebum and old dead skin. You can see them because the sebum has oxidized and turned black. Mind you, you cannot get to them easily, if at all, which can drive you crazy.

Whiteheads are *closed comedones*—all you see is a bump in the skin but no black content. It is really annoying to know that there is something under there but you cannot get to it. Please, do not try to squeeze them with your hands. You cannot push on the skin hard enough to get the sebum out. All you will accomplish is to get the site inflamed and red.

Please, do not let your local facialist try to clear your blackheads or whiteheads either. It does not work well. No amount of steaming the skin will open these plugged pores. And pinching can lead to infection and inflammation.

Instead of sheer force, we can apply some science to solve the problem. It stands to reason that if we abrade the skin first (as in microdermabrasion) or if we use a light chemical peel we will have an easier time.

Alternatively, we can apply some glycolic or salicylic acid peel first. As you know, these light acid peels (both AHA and BHA) loosen the "glue" that holds skin cells together and dissolve oily plugs (sebum) so you will have an easier time. The combination of light peels and microdermabrasion can literally "unroof" the blackheads or whiteheads so they come out more easily. However, even under ideal conditions, this will not happen after the first session. You will need quite a few sessions and you also have to do your exfoliation part at home to succeed.

I recently saw a twenty-four-year-old woman named Deirdre with an extensive whitehead/blackhead problem with many inflammatory acne sites. There was no evidence of deep cystic acne. She told me that her skin is very sensitive and she only uses gentle products. In fact, she used a cleanser that her mother had been using for years, and a night cream from the same source. "Any exfoliation?" I asked. "No, my skin is very sensitive, I'm afraid," she said.

The absence of deep cystic acne on her face was encouraging to me. It told me that the source of the problem might be her conviction that her skin is too sensitive for exfoliation. We did a series of combination salicylic peels and microdermabrasion treatments and put her on a very strict program of cleanser, toner, strong glycolic pads, and microdermabrasion cream for home use three times a week, along with topical antibiotics and Retin A. Her skin cleared to perfection within a few weeks.

A word of caution: once you have blackheads and whiteheads, it is unlikely that you can remove them all on your own in one sunny Sunday afternoon. It will take persistent work for quite a long time. You have to exfoliate with your serious-grade glycolic pads every night to make sure you do not go to bed with clogged pores, especially in the T-zone. The T-zone is the site of the heaviest oil production and therefore the most prone to acne outbreaks. You must use a microdermabrasion cream once or twice a week to further discourage clogged pores. If your skin is oily, use the cream three to four times per week. If you can, use a doctor's designed weekly AHA or BHA peel system. These are mostly preventive measures; you may not be able to get rid of all the blackheads already there.

If you can, have a doctor jump-start your skin with a series of superficial peels of glycolic, salicylic, lactic acid, a microdermabrasion series, or a combination of the two. Go on a short course of topical antibiotics (a serum). A doctor might even prescribe tretinoic acid (more on this later).

But keep things in perspective. Most of us are looking at our blackheads and whiteheads in a 3X mirror. Who else is looking at you that way? We all think that our blackheads and whiteheads are worse than they really are. If you exfoliate and care for your skin, blackheads and whiteheads will be treated effectively, and in most cases your face will clear.

INFLAMMATORY PUSTULES (AKA ACNE OR PIMPLES)

In some cases a clogged follicle with indwelling bacteria becomes infected and inflamed. It turns red and pustular and you have a classic acne breakout. This level of acne is still based mostly on clogged pores with bacterial invasion, as compared to the next level, which is deep, cystic acne. In deep, cystic acne, there may also be a hormonal component to the origin of the breakout.

From the perspective of prevention, first ask yourself one critical question: *Where is the breakout on my face?*

Why? Because sometimes acne can be self-induced. For example,

Anya is a twenty-seven-year-old female patient, built like a rock—she works out daily. She came to see me about recurring breakouts on her forehead. As I examined her face, I realized that there was no evidence of acne anywhere except on her forehead. If there were a hormonal cause to the acne, I would see acne on the chin first, and then on the cheeks. As we talked, I watched as she brushed her hair off her forehead. She told me that when she works out, she has to wear a bandanna to keep perspiration off her face.

This is a classic case of skin contamination from hands, hair, and the bandanna. The dirt and sweat don't cause acne, but they carry bacteria that, as we discussed earlier, settle into the sebum-rich clogged pores and cause acne. Your hair, your cell phone, a pencil, your own hands touching the face, all can easily contaminate the skin. I see so many patients with acne outbreaks on their forehead who have a habit of swiping hair off their face with their hands.

So ask yourself these questions: Where are my breakouts? Are my breakouts mostly near my hairline or on the forehead? Are bangs or a bandanna touching my skin? It is also possible to clog pores with hair spray or hair gel. Always cover your face when you apply these types of hair products.

Merrie came to see me with a fresh acne site on one side of her cheek. All the rest of her face was clear. There was just this one glaring group of outbreaks. I thought, if she had a tendency for acne, I would see it on the chin first before I see it on the cheek. I would also see some evidence of acne on the other cheek. Something just did not add up. I asked her to please pretend that she is making a phone call. Sure enough, the acne was where the phone touched her face. Another classic case of bacterial contamination.

If you wear glasses, do you get a breakout near the temple where you touch your face to take them off? When you read, write, take an exam, do you rest your head on your hands? Always look for the obvious first and keep in mind that *hands and objects should be kept off the face.*

CYSTIC ACNE (DEEP, PUSS-FILLED RED LUMPS UNDER THE SKIN)

In this most serious form of acne, the inflammation becomes so advanced that there is a deep, indwelling, puss-filled nodule under the skin, and a corresponding redness and even some pain on the skin surface. Deep cystic acne is most often on the chin or on the hollow of the cheeks and forehead. In deep cystic acne there is usually more to the cause than bacteria-infected, clogged sebaceous pores. There is an additional hormonal component.

Cystic acne usually begins in puberty as a consequence of a sudden surge of androgen hormones such as testosterone. Testosterone stimulates the sebaceous glands to produce oil, so much oil that it hopelessly clogs the pores, sometimes in spite of your best efforts.

Adult cystic acne is usually based on a hormonal cause as well. Some women get acne in perimenopause or menopause where there is a hormonal imbalance. Estrogen levels drop, which can allow for androgen hormone dominance.

Times of great stress can also cause a hormonal imbalance leading to a breakout. It isn't just your imagination that you break out at the worst times. Weddings, exam time, or job interviews are classic high-stress situations that could cause breakouts.

The hormonal changes of childbirth is another classic situation for deep cystic acne. After delivery, once hormonal balance is reestablished, in most cases the acne disappears by itself.

There is a famous infomercial on acne, one of the most successful ever. The commercial shows impressive before and after pictures. Maybe you've seen it. But have you noticed a remarkable trend in the testimonials? Most of the testimonials show glowingly happy *young mothers* with babies on their arms. The before picture was obviously taken while they were still pregnant or had just delivered. The after pictures were taken after the baby was born and the hormonal cause of acne subsided. Unfortunately, the television viewers who spend money on the product were unaware of the connection.

Deep cystic acne needs to be attended to by a doctor. Do not wait long to see him or her. The deeper the acne, the longer the red mark lasts afterward, and the more likely you could end up with a pitting scar.

Cystic acne needs to be treated by various means prescribed and administered by a doctor. We use:

- topical antibiotics

- oral antibiotics

- tretinoin-based creams (Retin A, Differin)

- oral tretinoin (Accutane) if all else fails

Light chemical peels (glycolic, salicylic acid) and microdermabrasion procedures help to jump-start your progress.

As far as what you do at home, try not to use any regular night creams meant for nonacne skin until the problem resolves. Make sure that any products you are using are noncomedogenic. Avoid petroleum jellylike products and old-fashioned creams that are filled with mineral oil—they can cause breakouts.

Do aggressive exfoliation; use glycolic cleansing pads; and only use thin, strong, water-based serums.

To hasten the resolution of acne, dermatologists sometimes inject the pustules with corticosteroids. This cure works well, but there is one possible grave complication: The shots can leave permanent depressions in the skin. This complication is what we call "operator-dependent." It is the function of how experienced your doctor is in injecting acne. You should not let nonmedical personnel inject corticosteroids into your acne site. And you should not be afraid to ask your doctor if that is a treatment he or she has often administered.

TREATING ACNE AT HOME WITH TOPICAL AND ORAL MEDICATION

Let us go over some potential pitfalls for starters.

If you suddenly develop whiteheads, blackheads, or acne, immediately ask yourself if you have changed your skin-care regimen, used a new makeup, or started some kind of treatment. If you have, stop and step up the exfoliation. I have seen so many young women in their twenties and thirties who were using heavy creams, much too occlusive for their age, and were giving themselves whiteheads and acne as a consequence.

If the outbreak is on your forehead or the side of the face, think about hair, baseball caps on a sweaty forehead, your hands, or hair sprays. If they are on the side of the face or chin, think about telephones and cell phones, your hands, pens, etc.

Also, think about the season. Few people realize that your summer skin care has to be different from your winter care or else at the end of summer you can wind up with more bumps under your skin. The dry, cold air during the winter or the winter dry heat requires heavier, more defensive skin care to protect your skin from drying out. However, if you keep using the same skin care into the hot and humid summer weather, you may cause pores to clog.

I was always very protective of my skin even as a young woman. Mind you, I did not always know what I was doing, as you will see. I remember before I went to medical school, I was using a night cream from one of the major department store brands that said right on the label that it was intended for mature skin. I was all of twenty-six at that time. But I thought if a little prevention is good, a lot of prevention is even better.

During the winter, all was well, but as soon as May came, I started to break out very badly. This was very unusual for me. I had no medical insurance and no money but I gathered whatever I had and went to a high-profile dermatologist. He injected the acne sites with corticosteroids during the course of an office visit that lasted no more than three minutes. As he and his nurse were racing out the door to see the next patient, the nurse turned around and said, "The cream you are using is too oily for your skin and for the summer season. Unless you change, you will be back for more injections, guaranteed." I felt like an idiot. How could I have missed that? Back then, of course, no one talked about exfoliation; this was even before glycolic acid was identified. But I took the nurse's advice and lightened up on the cream.

During the summer, use lighter creams and do not put any creams on the T-zone area. Use very little makeup during the day and make sure that the makeup you use is oil-free and noncomedogenic. Exfoliate more than usual using glycolic acid pads and make sure that you use an SPF 30 every day even if you are indoors, because exfoliation makes your skin slightly more vulnerable to sun damage.

As we review the roots of acne, we all realize the key role of exfoliation in the acne, whitehead/blackhead development process. AHA-based cleansing pads are remarkably important as a preventive measure because they help dissolve oily plugs and hasten the sloughing of dead old skin that, together with sebum, can potentially clog pores.

If you have acne, you should incorporate prescription acne products into your regimen as well. You need all the help you can get. Your doctor can prescribe topical antibiotic serums, which are an excellent choice. Tretinoin-based products such as Retin A and Differin regulate sebaceous release and exfoliate the skin. They are very helpful, as is topical benzoyl peroxide, which is an antimicrobial. The over-the-counter version is less effective than the prescription strength, but it is helpful.

A short course of oral antibiotic can be highly effective. I often prescribe minocycline, doxycycline, and erythromycin. If hormonal reasons appear to be part of the origin of the problem, low-dose birth control pills can be helpful.

If all these measures fail, including in-office treatments (see below), you may want to consider oral isotretinoin (Accutane). Accutane is highly effective, but should be used only as a last-ditch effort. The main issue with Accutane is that it is said to cause severe birth defects. Even several months after stopping the medication, there is a chance of birth defects. So if you are pregnant or likely to become pregnant, Accutane is not a good choice. Accutane's side effects, such as depression, even suicide, have received a lot of publicity recently. However, these side effects are extremely rare. If you take Accutane, liver function needs to be monitored regularly. It is a powerful medicine and can treat even the most severe deep cystic acne that nothing else can treat. But you must discuss this treatment very thoroughly with your doctor before you consider taking it.

TREATING ACNE AT THE DOCTOR'S OFFICE: PEELS, BLUE LIGHT, AND LASER TREATMENTS

Superficial glycolic acid peels are one of the most common peels to treat acne. Glycolic acid is an alpha-hydroxy acid in a peel form, which is usually given in combination with oral and topical medications. The peel reduces the amount of sebum trapped in the follicles and exfoliates dead skin. The peels are performed every two to four weeks in a series of four to eight sessions. If you are on prescription Retin A (or other tretinoic acid products), tell the doctor who performs the peel. You must stop using the drug for five days before you have the peel. Retin A can make the peel go much deeper than intended. If your acne is pregnancy-related, don't be concerned; glycolic acid products *are* considered safe for use during pregnancy.

Please note that if you are on oral Accutane, you cannot have light chemical peels or microdermabrasion because the peel may go too deep, with serious consequences. Please do not forget to mention to your doctor even if she or he forgets to ask.

Salicylic acid peels (salicylic acid is a beta-hydroxy acid, BHA for short) are also used to treat acne. Salicylic acid is oil-soluble, so it can more easily penetrate oil-plugged pores. The peel should be at least 20 to 30 percent acid. Otherwise it is not worth your time. Interestingly enough, salicylic acid peels are much safer than glycolic because they are self-limiting. They stop working by themselves. This is in contrast to glycolic acid peels that keep working on your face until you neutralize the acid. The longer the glycolic acid stays on your face, the deeper it goes. There is definitely a greater potential for error under these conditions. The salicylic acid peel, on the other hand, goes on your face, and in two to three minutes it stops working altogether. You can leave it on for any length of time (even by accident); it will not peel any farther than the first several minutes, so there is *no* potential for error. I use a combination of a 30 percent salicylic peel with microdermabrasion on acne patients with good success. A word of caution: many over-the-counter cleansers and toners make acne claims based on salicylic acid. By law you can only put a maximum of 2 percent salicylic acid in over-the-counter products. By now you know that is not enough to get results. So please do not spend much money on salicylic-containing over-the-counter products. The same 2 percent rule applies to all over-the-counter salicylic-acid-based creams or pads or lotions. For this reason, salicylic acid is rarely used by itself. It is usually combined with glycolic acid to enhance its effectiveness. Fortunately, glycolic acid can be found in higher concentrations in some products.

It is a shame that salicylic acid is limited to 2 percent by law because it is highly effective in higher doses and is remarkably safe, due to its self-limiting mechanism of action.

One new approach to treating acne is to target the bacteria that produce the inflammation. As you recall, the bacteria's name is *Propionobacterium acnes,* or *P. acnes. P. acnes* releases porphyrins. When porphyrins absorb certain wavelengths of light, free-radical damage is produced in them which, in turn, destroys the bacteria.

So how do you destroy porphyrins? Porphyrins absorb light in the blue color range (400 to 430 nm), so the treatment consists of a few sessions of low-intensity blue light. This is not a laser, it is simply blue light. It is only effective for mild to moderate inflammatory acne. *Why only mild to moderate acne?* Because severe acne most likely has a hormonal component as well. The blue light obviously has no effect on hormones.

A recent study shows that two fifteen-minute exposures a week for four weeks produced a 60 percent reduction in acne in 80 percent of patients. The remission time from acne lasted as long as three to eight months.

A new and very costly way to treat acne is using laser technology. The laser damages the sebaceous glands by heating them. The heat alters the sebaceous glands, which leads to a reduction of the amounts of oil produced. In a recent study, a 1,450 nm diode laser was used to perform four treatments one month apart. Six months later, there was 100 percent clearing of acne in sixteen of the seventeen patients evaluated.

My opinion is that laser for acne should be your last resort because of great expense. Try less expensive treatments such as glycolic and salicylic acid peels first. Use of lasers is not recognized by insurance companies as an acceptable treatment for acne, so financially you are on your own. If money is not an issue, the results can be very rewarding.

However, if your acne does not respond to laser treatment, do not stay with it for very long. My experience tells me that you will not respond to it successfully at a later time either—and your out-of-pocket expense will be considerable. A word of caution: if you are currently on Accutane or have been during the past six months, be sure to mention it to your doctor; otherwise your laser treatment or your peels may go too deep and cause major problems.

The laser can also be successful in reducing some of the redness associated with inflammation. Laser energy heats up the blood in the dilated vessels of the red area. In response, the blood coagulates and closes up the vessel. The now closed and nonfunctional vessels are reabsorbed and the inflammation disappears.

ACNE AND HORMONES

When adult women experience acne outbreaks, almost invariably hormones are to blame. Hormonal acne can be particularly difficult to treat because it does not respond to the same over-the-counter treatments that worked for you in the past.

Hormonally influenced acne usually begins in the early to midtwenties and can persist well into adulthood. Additionally, it can reemerge around the time of perimenopause or menopause. The cause of hormonal acne is linked to androgens, male hormones that stimulate the sebaceous oil glands in the skin. If sebaceous glands are overstimulated by androgens, acne can occur. Nearly half of all women experience acne outbreaks and increased facial oiliness during the week prior to menstruation.

Most women with acne have normal androgen levels; however, some women may have a more serious medical condition for which acne is just one symptom. Polycystic ovary disease and adrenal hyperplasia are two of those conditions where persistent cystic acne prevails. These conditions are associated with many other symptoms, such as significant facial hair, loss of hair from the scalp, irregular menstrual cycle, obesity, infertility, and diabetes. If you have a cluster of these symptoms, prompt medical attention is essential.

TREATING HORMONAL ACNE

Treating hormonal acne is a difficult problem. The treatment options include topical retinoids, topical antimicrobials (such as benzoyl peroxide and antibiotics), and oral antibiotics that are prescribed when the inflammation is severe.

For women with hormonal acne who develop premenstrual outbreaks, oral contraceptive pills (OCPs) can be used successfully. OCPs contain estrogen and progestin. They regulate the menstrual cycle and decrease the androgen activity responsible for acne, leading to decreased breakouts. Another medication that may be prescribed in conjunction with an oral contraceptive is spironolactone, an anti-androgen. Spironolactone prevents excessive oil production by blocking androgen receptors and decreasing androgen production in both the ovaries and adrenal glands.

While OCPs are effective in treating hormonal acne, they can cause side effects. Mild side effects, which usually subside after the first month or two after starting the medication, include breast tenderness, bloating, and nausea. However, more serious complications, such as blood clots or strokes, do occur, although they are now less common with the newer formulations that contain less estrogen. My opinion is to try your hardest to prevent and treat acne topically first, before you resort to OCPs.

Pregnant women often experience bouts of acne, but, of course, treatment options are limited due to potential penetration of active medication through the skin. Topical antibiotics are usually prescribed.

Postmenopausal acne is also common due to a decrease in estrogen levels and the relative increase of androgenic hormones. Fortunately, traditional acne therapies, as well as anti-androgens, are good treatment options.

ROSACEA

Rosacea is a chronic and often progressive skin disease that causes redness and swelling on the face. Rosacea is a condition similar to acne and is often confused with acne, but it has a different source and treatment. Rosacea may include acnelike outbreaks on occasion, but the key feature that describes rosacea is dilated red visible capillaries that actually gave the name rosacea (*rosa* for red). As many as 14 million people in the United States have rosacea, most between ages thirty and fifty. It is most common in fair-skinned individuals. (A side note: broken capillaries are *not* specific only to rosacea.) Rosacea may first manifest itself as a tendency to flush easily. After a while it progresses to persistent redness in the center of the face. It may gradually involve the cheeks, nose, forehead, and chin. As the disease progresses, the redness becomes more severe and persistent. The small, superficial blood vessels, acnelike outbreaks, and red nodules become permanently visible. Rosacea can be exacerbated by sunlight, hot drinks, alcohol, spicy foods, extremes of hot and cold temperature, and emotional stress.

In the treatment of rosacea the first step is to avoid the known exacerbating factors noted above. The medical therapy of rosacea includes oral and topical antibiotics.

Glycolic acid peels are often used in conjunction with antibiotics to bring about an improvement in the condition. After a peel you may be red for a few hours, but please do not use makeup during this time. A series of peels are performed every two to four weeks and may be used in combination with low-concentration glycolic acid washes and creams.

Topical or oral therapies may resolve the acnelike component of rosacea; however, they do not remove the redness or reduce the appearance of dilated blood vessels associated with rosacea.

However, vascular lasers and intense pulsed light source (similar to laser equipment) can successfully address the dilated blood vessels. They are very successful in improving the appearance of redness in rosacea.

Vascular lasers emit specific wavelengths of light targeted for the tiny visible blood vessels just under the skin. Heat from the laser's energy builds in the vessels, causing them to collapse. The newest generation of vascular lasers does not produce any bruising, but may cause redness and minimal swelling that lasts approximately twenty-four to forty-eight hours.

Intense light and laser therapy use multiple wavelengths of light to treat dilated blood vessels in the face. Both treatments, laser and intense light, use laser sources. The session takes fifteen to thirty minutes and needs to be repeated every six weeks for a total of four to six times. Of course, the number of sessions is variable. Patients may require several treatments initially, and may return annually for treatment of new blood vessels.

You know I am the last one to tell you to spend your hard-earned money on lasers, but these methods work. There are no good alternative treatment options in treating facial redness other than these lasers.

A word of caution: make sure that you go only to a qualified physician for vascular laser treatment. Never trust a spa or even a medical spa where there is no qualified physician present. Lasers can burn and cause permanent damage.

A spa may claim that it has a laser for rosacea; however, spas are not allowed, by law, to own a proper medical-grade laser that actually makes a difference. They may own a laser, and the laser salesman may have told them that it treats rosacea, so they may not be lying to you. However, there is a world of difference between a low-output laser that a spa may be allowed to own, and a high-output medical laser in terms of results. It is much like the difference between a toy telephone and the real one. High-output lasers are dangerous machinery; they belong in a qualified physician's office only. I will never forget K.H., a beautiful twenty-nine-year-old girl of Middle Eastern ancestry, who came to my office with remarkably disfiguring dark and light spots on her face. She told me she had some red acne scars. She went to a spa where she was told that a vascular laser could successfully heal these red scars. She even asked, "Do you have a supervising doctor?" "Oh, yes, we do" was the answer. The technician used settings much too high for her Middle Eastern complexion. Now she has permanent pigment loss (white spots) and significant hyperpigmentation in the treated area. I suppose the doctor, if there in fact was a doctor, was off that day. A terrible shame. Interestingly enough, if your skin is very light, the chance that anything can go wrong with vascular lasers is minimal. Darker skins, however, are much less forgiving. If the laser energy is set too high for your skin type, you can end up with disfiguring dark and hypopigmented (light) discolorations. If you have darker skin (Italian,

Greek, Turkish, Middle Eastern, Spanish, African ancestry), please be especially careful.

In advanced cases of rosacea, rhinophyma may develop, a condition that occurs when oil glands enlarge on the face and a bulbous, enlarged red nose and swollen cheeks develop. This relatively rare condition usually occurs in men over forty. The excess tissue can be surgically removed using lasers, dermabrasion, or electrosurgery to sculpt the nose back down to a more normal shape and appearance.

Telangiectasia, little red capillaries under the skin, can also be successfully treated by vascular lasers based on the same principle of heat closing the blood vessels. Treatments need to be repeated four to six times at four- to six-week intervals. Individual needs may vary greatly.

ACNE SCARS

By far, the worst part of acne is the aftermath: the scars. As you know, acne is an inflammatory condition, so if we study the natural history of acne, we learn about the natural course of the inflammatory process.

The three stages are:

1. *The red stage.* Redness, node under the skin, some pain at times, then puss and some more redness that persists, sometimes for weeks or months.

2. *The dark stage.* Next comes the postinflammatory hyperpigmentation stage, when dark pigment cells (melanocytes) march in and turn the former red spot into a persistent darker spot. If you have a little more pigment in your skin (Mediterranean, Latin, African-American), you may have dark spots at former acne sites that persist for months or years.

3. *The pitting stage.* If the inflammation process is beyond a certain magnitude, tight scar tissue forms and pulls the skin down, giving rise to dreaded pitting scars, that are permanent.

Acne would be almost tolerable if it came one day, culminated into a pustular head in three days, and then disappeared as if it were never there. This is not what happens. Acne comes, culminates in a breakout, and then redness lingers for weeks to months. The lighter your skin, the longer it lingers as a bright red spot just to remind you who is the boss. The deeper the acne cyst, the longer the redness persists. I have patients who can show me painful reminders of an outbreak that occurred six months earlier. If you are older, the redness lingers longer than it used to. If you have some color in your skin, you will develop a dark spot. The darker you are, the deeper the color, and the longer the spots will last.

Vascular lasers are really handy at the red stage. If you can desiccate the blood vessels, the red spot can readily disappear. This is key because by interrupting the blood supply, you may shorten the natural history of the inflammatory process, avoiding the dark stage and the possible pitting stage. The longer the red inflammatory stage persists, the more likely that a dark, hyperpigmented spot will develop in its place. The length of time of the red stage is critical.

Unfortunately, vascular lasers are too dangerous for darker skins because dark skins hyperpigment easily. The reason is that the laser looks for a color contrast. It can focus on a red color with a white background or a dark color with a white background. Without proper contrast, the laser can burn both the target area and the background. That's the last thing we want.

The latest treatment options for acne scarring are lasers such as the pulsed carbon dioxide (CO_2) laser and the erbiumYAG laser.

The CO_2 laser vaporizes thin layers of the skin and tightens collagen fibers, which makes it an appropriate treatment for depressed acne scars. The erbiumYAG laser vaporizes thinner layers and produces very precise bursts of energy, which allows for the sculpting of smaller, irregular scars. CO_2 laser-treated skin heals in seven to ten days, while erbiumYAG laser-treated sites heal in three to five days.

However, laser resurfacing is not always effective for acne scars. The depressed, craterlike scars are hardest to deal with. An option for improving the appearance of these scars is soft-tissue augmentation. That means that the craterlike scars are filed until they are no longer noticeable. Patients can opt to use their own fat from another part of the body to correct the deep contour, or they can use soft-tissue fillers such as collagen, hyaluronic acid, or fascia lata. This treatment typically lasts six to eighteen months and then has to be redone.

All of these treatments are expensive and uncomfortable. The real key to treating acne is to cut back on the inflammatory stage, because this is when the trouble starts. If we can tame the inflammatory process at the very beginning, we can avoid the persistent redness, the ensuing darkness, and the possible pitting scar tissue. The question is: how?

Good skin care and hygiene help. A healthier, less stressful lifestyle plays a part.

One of my personal secrets for treating my occasional acne outbreaks is to put a prescription-strength corticosteroid cream on the cystic acne site at the earliest sign of an outbreak. I cover it with a bandage strip to keep it on all night, because without coverage (occlusion) it does not work. By the morning, the acne has usually shrunk. I repeat this once or twice before the acne is gone. Ever since I began this method, I have not had a red acne scar. I still break out from time to time, but the acne does not have a chance to survive on my face. There you have it. I am taking a real chance by giving you my secret because this is far from any accepted acne therapies. The danger is that prolonged steroid use on skin thins out the skin, so one must limit this treatment to one to two nights only. This treatment has a similar effectiveness to corticosteroid injection into the acne site, but, of course, it's less risky!

The ultimate solution to the acne problem would be to treat the skin with a highly effective, nonsteroidal, anti-inflammatory agent. With a nonsteroidal agent, we could cut back on the severity of the inflammatory stage significantly without running the risk of thinning the skin. Research is discovering some of these agents. One of them, phytosphyngosine, is already available. I have built this agent into a sticky acne patch that you put on the acne site overnight. It is remarkably effective! These patches are very popular among my patients.

If you had acne and oily skin as a teenager, you never recover from the fear of acne. You struggle with occasional, hormone-related acne most of your life. Then in your forties, you start to notice that your dry-skinned, acne-free contemporaries look older and more wrinkled than you do. There is a justice in this, I suppose, although if you ask the acne sufferer, she is usually not ready to admit it. Scars of acne run deep. Luckily, there is so much more we can do about acne these days.

CHAPTER NINE

DR. DENESE'S QUICK FIXES FOR SKIN EMERGENCIES

The love of your life from twenty-five years ago called, he is now divorced, like you, and wants to see you for the first time next Tuesday. . . . Your thirty-year high school reunion is coming up in two weeks. . . . You are going on job interviews after ten years of staying at home. . . . Your daughter is getting married in a few months. . . . There can be so many reasons why you suddenly feel you have to look good, or better than usual. What do you do?

How can you get ready for a special occasion and look more radiant than your usual self if you have only three months? Or three weeks? Or just three days?

Don't panic. There are ways to make yourself look much better even if you only have three days or even three hours. (Although if you only have three minutes, I am not sure I can help you!)

THE THREE-DAY QUICK FIX

Let's start with the worst-case scenario. You are getting ready for a major occasion—like your wedding, for instance—and three days before the event you get a huge breakout on your chin. It's so bad that you can't even cover it. What do you do? This is a beauty emergency if I ever saw one.

If you have an experienced dermatologist, you can have the outbreak injected by a minuscule amount of corticosteroid, which will force the acne to recede by the next day. *If* you get an appointment, *if* you have the time to go there, *if* you have a dermatologist, or *if* you can find one in time . . . there are too many "ifs" here to make me feel comfortable. If you can, go to a dermatologist, but if there is no way you can get to one, you can do the following.

Take a prescription-strength corticosteroid cream and put a fair amount on the acne itself, at night. Now comes the most important step: Take a Band-Aid, but cut off the gauze part so it doesn't absorb the cream, and use the sticky part only to cover the cream for the entire night. If the cream is a strong enough corticosteroid, you will see dramatic shrinkage of the breakout by the morning. You cannot—and I repeat, you *cannot*—do this more than two to three days in a row on one area because corticosteroids thin the skin and can cause other problems. Corticosteroids are excellent in reducing the acute inflammation involved with acne, but they thin your skin in the long run, which can be detrimental. This is also *not* a good method if you have many outbreaks or frequent outbreaks. If you do, you need a treatment that addresses the problem itself and not just the symptoms. However, this method is ideal for the occasional acne outbreak that comes at a bad time.

Here's a quick tip if you have swollen, baggy eyes. Treat the condition by applying ice a few hours before you have to go out. The ice will bring the puffiness down at least for the evening. However, if you have more time, you deserve a better solution. Under-eye bags are worth a visit to a reputable plastic surgeon because they are most often caused by a fat pad. Dealing with the fat pad is a relatively easy surgical procedure, which can make a big improvement in your looks and requires a short recovery time.

If you have more visible lines around the eyes than you would like, buy yourself a collagen or vitamin C eye patch that is intended to be left on the skin all night. The occlusion and the ingredients will cause a slight cosmetic plumping of the skin, so you can look better the next day. The effect is temporary, but we take what we can get at times.

If you have a week to deal with the lines before your event, I recommend a Botox injection. It takes at least four to five days until Botox takes full effect, but there is no question that it makes a remarkable difference in the depth and number of lines around the eyes.

For overall skin vitality, try to have a light microdermabrasion process three days before the event. It will give you a noticeable glow and radiance. On the other hand, I would not recommend a glycolic acid, salicylic acid, or fruit acid peel three days before an important event. You might still be red and peeling after only three days. If you have a week, by all means get one.

You can get an oxygen facial in a spa or a spa facial, as well. It may give you a beautiful glow for the evening. Do this right before the event, though, because the effect does not last. If you have a choice between microdermabrasion or an oxygen facial, I would probably choose the microdermabrasion because it is slightly more invasive and you may get more benefits out of it. If you aren't strapped for money, you can have both. Remember, the more invasive the procedure, the better the outcome—even within the category of light, office-based peels. If you have a choice between a spa facial and a medical spa or doctor's office light peel, I would choose the medical spa or the doctor's treatment.

If you have no time or availability for a professional peel, do not despair. I rarely have time to get one either, so welcome to the club. We just have to work extra hard with our home-based exfoliants to achieve that certain radiant glow. Your pads and your microdermabrasion cream should get an extra workout. The night before I have to go on television, I use a strong cosmetic AHA/BHA cosmetic peel with vitamin C, and I get many positive comments about my skin.

THE THREE-WEEK QUICK FIX

If you have three weeks, you can do quite a bit more. You may have the time for some soft-tissue filler injections as well. If you are troubled by deep nasolabial folds or marionette lines at the corners of the mouth, three weeks is enough time to get the filler injections and recover if you have any swelling or bruising. Filler injections can often make you slightly swollen for two days after the injections, and you can have some bruising as well. It pays to give yourself a small cushion of time for recovery.

I would do Botox injections three weeks in advance for the same reason.

You may want to consider a temporary lip-enhancing injection as well. But you also need at least three weeks in case of bruising.

No matter what you decide about fillers or Botox, you still have to take care of the skin surface. If you can, treat yourself to one or two light, in-office peels before the big event. If that's not possible, you have to step up use of your at-home skin exfoliating arsenal. Use your microdermabrasion creams at least twice a week and use an over-the-counter peel.

If you struggle with red capillaries on your cheeks or even rosacea, three weeks is enough time to improve the condition, or at least start the process and have some visible improvement by the end of the third week. You need to visit a reputable doctor or a medical spa equipped with a vascular laser. The effect of a vascular laser on capillaries and even on redness associated with rosacea is evident in a day or two. You may repeat the process for even better results, and you still can stay within your time budget.

THE THREE-MONTH QUICK FIX

There's a lot you can do in three months. My six-step program will show you noticeable changes in eight weeks. And three months gives you enough time to go for the peels and procedures we discussed in chapter 7, the consultation chapter.

If you have three months, try to sign up for a series of light peels. You may even have time for a medium peel but not for a deep peel.

I have a lot of mothers of brides who seek me out a few weeks before the wedding, looking for a solution that may give a slight lift to the face without surgery. I often suggest a nonsurgical procedure that can do this temporarily. It is done by electrically stimulating facial muscles to contract many times during a session, which gives a dramatic lifted appearance to the face. You need about ten to twelve sessions twice a week to achieve a dramatic result. The effect is based on tightening the facial musculature so the result will stay with you only if you keep maintaining the effect. The procedure is expensive and time-consuming, but, of course, this does not keep the Hollywood crowd from using the procedure. Many movie stars use these sessions to try to look younger for a part if there is no time for surgery.

The same procedure can be performed for the body as well. These electrodes can build up muscles remarkably well and fast, which can supplement your exercise program.

Suppose you are getting ready for the summer. Wouldn't it be nice not to have to struggle with bikini, underarm, or leg hair? Three months will give you enough time to reduce your hair growth on a long-lasting or even on a permanent basis with laser hair removal. A few important pointers. You need to be as light-skinned as possible for laser hair removal to be effective. A trace of suntan will undermine your results. The procedure works best with dark hair, because the laser is based on contrast. (Suntan and light hair decrease the contrast.) The dark pigments of the hair pick up the laser energy and burn. The idea is that by overheating the hair follicle, it becomes disabled and will not be able to sprout more hair. It is best to choose a laser that goes deep into the hair follicle because this may give you the best chance for long-term change. Ask your doctor about the depth of penetration of his particular laser. Remember: lasers cannot remove blond hair effectively because the lack of dark pigment in blond hair does not allow for absorption of sufficient laser energy to overheat the follicles.

Many of my patients complain of a sudden surge of coarse facial hair after menopause. Dark facial hair can be removed by laser. One word of caution: try to remove it as soon as you can. If you wait a few years and the hairs turn white, lasers can do nothing to remove them because of lack of pigmentation. In that case, your only option is electrolysis.

Three months is enough time to turn a new page in your at-home skin care and place it on a more scientific basis. You may see positive changes in as little as a month's time, which leaves you two more months to achieve further benefits.

Come to think of it, three months is a very handy deadline to start implementing some of the anti-aging measures we have discussed in this book. If you have three months to get ready, you can do some significant inside as well as outside preparations. This is a perfect opportunity to go on a new diet and combine it with an exercise program that you follow religiously for three months. You can start a new vitamin supplementation program complete with some of the key vitamins and nutrients we discussed in chapter 3. Three months is long enough to see some noticeable results.

It is difficult to make the commitment "from now until forever," but it is not so hard to give yourself a three-month deadline and carefully follow through with the commitments you have made for yourself. So let's not wait for a special occasion; let's get started right now to feel better and look younger as soon as we can.

CHAPTER TEN

DR. DENESE'S SHOPPING GUIDE

Step through the front door of many of the biggest and best department stores in America and what do you see? Counter after counter of cosmetics products. If you are like many of the patients I meet in my practice, you may feel overwhelmed by all the choices that confront you. Which products are worth your money? Which jars and bottles will deliver on their promises, and which will disappoint you after you've spent your hard-earned dollars and brought them home, only to find after a few weeks of use that they did nothing to improve the condition of your skin? How do you know exactly what you are putting on your face? What works? What doesn't? How can you avoid being fooled by empty and deceptive promises?

There are no easy answers to these questions. The label on the product *should* tell you everything you need to know, but anyone who has ever looked at a label on a jar of cream or a bottle of cleanser knows that it is written in the language of chemistry. The ingredients are listed in descending order, starting with the ingredient present in the highest percentage. That's pretty clear, but unfortunately the ingredients are listed using their chemical names. This makes it very hard to understand what is actually inside the jar or bottle.

The Food and Drug Administration (FDA), which began monitoring cosmetics in 1938, realizes that most consumers do not understand the chemical names of the ingredients, but there is no way to remedy this problem. The ingredients can only be accurately described by their scientific names because there are no common names for them.

Despite the highly technical language, you do not have to be a cosmetics scientist to get valuable information off the label. (On pages 181–88 I've included a translation guide, explaining the names of ingredients to look for as well as some to look *out* for.) If you are armed with a few basic definitions and an understanding of just how the cosmetics industry uses legally worded puffery to sell its products, it is possible to decode cosmetics labels and be a savvy shopper.

FACT VS. FICTION

All cosmetics, whether sold in retail stores or through a salon or doctor's office, are subject to the Food, Drug, and Cosmetic Act. This law mandates that the product label must state the name and place of business (city, state, and Zip code) of the manufacturer, packer, or distributor, the quantity of the contents, and any appropriate directions for safe use and/or warning statements. Additional regulations require that all ingredients be listed on the label by their scientific name.

What the law does *not* require is a listing of the percentage content of the ingredients because, if the percentages were shown, anyone could replicate the product. Cosmetics formulas are, in fact, closely guarded secrets, often kept in a safe by the owner.

Few people realize that most small- to medium-size cosmetics companies do not own their products' formulas. In most cases, the companies place an order for a formula with one of the handful of cosmetics manufacturing factories in the United States, requesting, for instance, "an eye cream with vitamin C." The manufacturer then either has its chemistry lab develop a new formula, or it borrows an old formula from its past inventory and presents it for the client's approval. If the product meets the company's criteria, the manufacturer fills the order. If not, it's back to the lab to try again until approval is obtained.

Large companies, such as Lancôme and Estée Lauder, have their own labs, but very few small cosmetics companies go to the trouble and expense of employing chemists and developing their own formulas. So if you think you have experienced a particular eye cream before, you may not be imagining it. The same cream could come from one manufacturer's lab, simply wearing a different label. I am unusual because I hired my own chemist when I decided to develop a product line. Many of my colleagues in the industry thought this decision would drive me into financial hardship, but I believed it was the most important place to invest. Simply put, if you have your own chemist, you own your formulations. If you do not own the formulations, then the manufacturer can sell the identical recipe to someone else. This idea troubled me so much that I decided that having my own chemist was essential, so all my products can be unique to me and conform to my ideas of what works.

In some instances the percentage of an ingredient may be listed in the front of a product, right under the name. But if it's there, it's voluntary, and it is done to impress you, the buyer. A prime example is vitamin C. In many of the good, doctor-brand vitamin C serums, you will see the percentage displayed prominently on the front (10 percent vitamin C in SkinCeuticals, for instance). In fact, if you see a vitamin C serum that does not proclaim the vitamin percentage on the front panel, you can assume that the percentage is in the low single digits, and the product may be less helpful to your skin.

WHAT IS A COSMETIC?

According to the FDA, a cosmetic is a product that is applied to the skin for cleansing, beautifying, and promoting attractiveness or altering the appearance of the skin. But sometimes a cosmetic is a drug as well, and then it falls under different labeling regulations altogether.

There are three main cosmetic/drug items:

- sunscreens

- acne treatment products

- skin-fading (dark-skin-discoloration-fading) products

You may have noticed that a drug fact label box always appears on the back of every size and variety of these products. The FDA requires it, and also has strict rules about the exact wording and punctuation that must be used. This is why all labels look and sound alike. The percentage of the active ingredients is required on a drug fact label, so you can know exactly how much zinc oxide or titanium dioxide is in your sunscreen; how much hydroquinone is contained in your skin fader cream; and how strong an acne-fighting effect you can expect from a skin pad, scrub, or cream.

Any product with a drug fact label needs to go through strictly regulated effectiveness testing to be sure that it does what it claims to do. These products must be tested in an FDA-approved independent testing facility and manufactured in an FDA-approved facility. This is important for you to know because when you go to the beach, you have to be certain that you can trust your skin to that small bottle of sunscreen in your beach bag.

The situation with all other cosmetics products is, unfortunately, not so clear.

WHAT'S IN A WORD?

A lot less than you imagine, especially when it comes to describing what a skin-care preparation can do for you. Unlike sunscreens, skin faders, and acne products, there are generally no percentages stated on the bottle or jar to help you assess which product would be better or more valuable for you. Essentially you are left to use your own judgment.

If you turn to the back of the bottle you cannot count on much more help. The wording on the bottle is very carefully regulated to comply with strict legal requirements. For instance, it cannot say that it "makes the skin younger." On the other hand, it *can* say it "makes the skin visibly younger" or makes the skin "younger-looking." In the same vein, a label cannot say that a product "will prevent aging," but it can claim to "prevent the appearance of aging" or "prevent the signs of aging." As long as qualifiers such as "visibly" and "the appearance of" are present, the statements comply with the law. The only time a product can be called a "skin fader" is if it contains hydroquinone. All other skin-lightening agents must be referred to as skin lighteners or brighteners, but not as faders.

PRODUCT SAFETY AND EFFICACY TESTING

PRODUCT SAFETY

Whether driven by altruism, liability, or the bottom line, most companies test their products for safety. The products are tested on about fifty to a hundred people for allergic reactions. From a scientific perspective, this is a large enough testing sample from which to draw conclusions; however, there may still be individuals who will have an allergic reaction. If it happens to you, stop using the product and do not experiment any further.

To remain impartial, the cosmetics companies do not test the products themselves. They hire one of a few independently owned cosmetics testing companies to run their tests. (The same ones are used by almost everyone in the industry.) In this way the results are objective and reliable.

All reputable companies have a lot at stake when it comes to safety, and they test their products regularly. As a matter of course, QVC requires safety testing on every cosmetics product it sells. I know, because I appear on QVC to sell my products. Companies on the Internet may or may not submit their products for allergy testing because it costs a lot and it is not easy to arrange for allergy testing.

When the product goes through safety testing, it can be marketed with the claim that it is "allergy tested," "hypoallergenic," "dermatologist tested," "sensitivity tested," or "nonirritating." Not all manufacturers put these claims on the bottle, even if the product is tested, but they keep the test results on file, for self-protection, in the rare case that something goes wrong with a consumer.

EFFICACY TESTING

Efficacy testing is very different from safety testing. While nearly all products go through safety testing, fewer products go through efficacy testing. These tests look for favorable changes that occur in the skin after a few weeks of use, such as reduction of wrinkles, improvement in the tightness of the skin, the look of pores, skin hydration, and moisture level. For the sake of impartiality, efficacy testing must be conducted in an independent testing lab, one that is owned by an independent company.

The best, most reliable skin-care testing produces results from measuring skin improvements with instruments that quantify the changes numerically. If a product can generate significant numerical changes, a company is allowed to print that information on the packaging. For example, a claim such as "87% improvement in skin hydration in two weeks." The law requires that every numerical claim be backed by an efficacy study.

Very few new cosmetics products generate measurable changes great enough to merit printing on the package. A 3 to 8 percent increase in hydration will hardly excite consumers. Most efficacy studies within the cosmetics industry end up at the bottom of a filing cabinet, while the high cost of conducting them becomes a tax deduction. But have you ever seen advertisements that boldly state something like "an independent consumer testing survey shows 87% of women experience an improvement in their skin. . . ."? Sounds impressive, doesn't it? Advertising copywriters are hoping that is just how you'll respond. They want you to believe that the product can bring about great changes for you, too, and they'd like you to think they are reporting a scientific, numerical measurement resulting from an efficacy study. But beware: they are not! This is just one more trick that the cosmetics industry uses that I want you to know about.

When a product is submitted for efficacy testing, the lab measures the skin changes after four to eight weeks of application. Scientific instruments are used to generate hard scientific data. But, at the same time, the testing facility also gathers study participants and gives them questionnaires to answer. If the instrumental data do not show any respectable changes, the "soft data" compiled from the questionnaires may. Indeed, this is usually the case: the study participants or the "trained observers" working for the testing company are more likely to say something positive about the product than the cold scientific instrument. You guessed it: the company uses the data from the questionnaires—the data that show better numbers. Let's say the scientific instrument showed a 6 percent increase in skin moisture content. On the other hand, 78 percent of the study participants said there was an improvement in skin moisture—whether it was a 6 percent or a 20 percent improvement, *it was an improvement*. If 78 percent of the participants agreed there was an improvement (a little or a lot), the package or advertising will use the 78 percent number—not the 6 percent.

THE POWER OF VITAMINS

At any cosmetics counter, you're sure to see many products that make a big issue of the fact that they contain vitamins. And there is no doubt about it: vitamins can provide great benefits when applied to your skin. But there are many considerations that determine if a product will use vitamins in a way that makes them truly effective. It's not only which vitamins are used, but also the concentration and the pH level (acidity) as well as the delivery method that determine if a product works.

At the center of any discussion of vitamins in skin-care products is vitamin C. Vitamin C (l-ascorbic acid) is one of the relatively few topical agents whose effectiveness against wrinkles is backed by reliable scientific evidence. One of the key figures who deserves a great deal of credit for vitamin C clinical studies is Dr. Mustafa Omar, who pioneered the vitamin C efficacy studies along with Dr. Sheldon Pinnell from Duke University.

In theory, vitamin C can benefit the skin in two important ways. First, vitamin C is an essential ingredient for collagen synthesis. Collagen, as you know, is responsible for the elasticity of the skin. If you add vitamin C to a petri dish with fibroblasts (skin cells that make collagen), you see a dramatic increase in collagen production. Second, vitamin C is a key antioxidant that can protect you from free-radical damage that comes from sun exposure or any other source. So if vitamin C is properly delivered into the skin at the right strength, the potential benefits are remarkable.

However, most medium- or less expensively priced vitamin C serums do not work. The reasons are insufficient concentrations and lack of stability.

Only highly concentrated preparations (10 percent or more)

deliver enough vitamin C to be topically effective. Beware of any vitamin C products that do not list the amount of vitamin C on the front label. If no percentage is listed, it's likely the percentage is below 10 percent.

The second problem is stability. When exposed to air, vitamin C undergoes oxidation. The oxidized form of vitamin C is not only incapable of boosting collagen synthesis and scavenging free radicals, but it actually *causes* free-radical damage to skin proteins. The l-ascorbic acid form of vitamin C is the best-penetrating but the *least* stable form of vitamin C. All the published studies that established vitamin C's success against wrinkles were conducted using l-ascorbic acid. Today some manufacturers ignore these facts, use other forms of vitamin C, and then ride on the coattails of the original vitamin C studies.

A few skin-care companies offer highly concentrated l-ascorbic acid vitamin C that is supposed to be stabilized and effective. Cellex C High Potency Serum and SkinCeuticals C & E and Serum 20 are among these. The prices they command are remarkably high, and even these products are not immune to the stability problem. In fact, not long ago, Cellex C received a lot of negative media coverage because of serums that turned dark and oxidized while still on the store shelves. Once vitamin C oxidizes, it is useless.

The oxidized vitamin C is dark yellow to brown. A fresh vitamin C serum is colorless. Brown tint usually indicates oxidation. Interestingly enough, manufacturers often add a yellow color to their vitamin C serum so it becomes hard to tell the state of oxidation. Perhaps the best way to get around this problem is use a "do it yourself" vitamin C serum kit, where you add the vitamin C powder to a serum right before the serum gets used.

Even when using an optimal and stable formulation of vitamin C, not everyone's skin will respond. Only about half of the users show noticeable benefits. Others may respond to vitamin C derivatives. Ascorbyl palmitate is one of these derivatives; it is the most widely used fat-soluble derivative of vitamin C. However, please beware, *it is not nearly*

GETTING YOUR DAILY DOSE OF VITAMINS IN SKIN CARE

Ingredient	Benefits
VITAMIN A	Helps stimulate the renewal of new skin cells and tissue. Used to treat dry skin, age spots, acne, sun damage. Also helps minimize the appearance of pore size and reduce the appearance of fine lines and wrinkles.
VITAMIN B	A moisturizer often used to repair damaged hair, with similar conditioning properties when applied to the skin.
VITAMIN C	An antioxidant that promotes the production of collagen and maintains skin's suppleness and elasticity.
VITAMIN D	An antioxidant that regulates cell turnover and helps control psoriasis.
VITAMIN E	In medical setting it was shown to accelerate wound healing, to combat dry skin, and help prevent untraviolet light damage.
VITAMIN F	An essential fatty acid.
VITAMIN K	In a clinical study it was shown to diminish the appearance of under-eye circles and bruises; fat-soluble.

Also known as	Additional info
In prescription form it's known as tretinoic acid or branded as Retin A or Renova. Its chemically-related non-prescription form is retinol.	The prescription-strength is often irritating. Tolerance must be built up over time, but effectiveness is excellent. It is the most widely used agent in the war against wrinkles. Causes increased sun sensitivity; SPF 30 protection used with it every day is essential. Not to be used if pregnant or nursing.
Biotin, Panthenol (provitamin B_5)	Often found in high-end serums.
L-ascorbic acid, ascorbyl palmitate, magnesium ascorbyl phosphate, and vitamin C ester	Widely available in skin-care products. The most difficult vitamin to stabilize. Once it oxidizes and darkens, it loses its potency as an antioxidant; then stop using it.
Branded as Dovonex, in prescription form.	Found in many commercial creams in small quantities.
Alpha tocopherol, tocopheryl acetate, and tocopheryl linoleate	Remarkably important ingredient. Fat-soluble only. In cosmetics products it's key to find it in high enough percentages to be effective. Often incorporated into sunscreens.
Linoleic acid, omega 3, EPA linolenic acid, evening primrose oil, black currant, flaxseed oil	Highly effective lipid even in small percentages to re-create skin lipid barrier.
Can be derived from the synthetic compound menadione (sometimes called vitamin K_3).	Extremely expensive raw material, which means that it is difficult to find a product that contains a high enough percentage of it to be effective.

as effective in building collagen as l-ascorbic acid or magnesium ascorbyl phosphate.

Magnesuim ascorbyl phosphate is a water-soluble derivative of vitamin C. It has the same potential in building collagen as l-ascorbic acid; however, it is much more stable and less irritating. L-ascorbic acid, the original vitamin C, needs to be in a highly acidic environment to be effective, which adds to the irritation. There are many skin care products on the market with magnesium ascorbyl phosphate, but their percentage falls well under the effective minimum dose needed for skin collagen stimulation. The reason is that magnesium ascorbyl phosphate is very expensive—far more expensive than l-ascorbic acid. The price is so high that it startles any manufacturer. Therefore, magnesium ascorbyl phosphate is a prime candidate for "angel dusting." Remember angel dusting? It is the practice of putting just a minimal amount of an expensive ingredient into the formulation, just to be able to list it on the label.

There is one more form of vitamin C in the market: vitamin C ester, which is more stable and less irritating. However, more clinical studies are needed to prove its clinical efficacy.

Fortunately, the situation with all the remaining vitamins is less controversial and less complicated. The central issue with the rest of vitamins is the manufacturing cost. High-potency vitamin products come with relatively high price tags. Also, as you may recall, the best way to deliver vitamins is in a thin, water-consistency serum as opposed to a cream. A much higher percentage of the vitamin will be absorbed from a thin serum than from a cream. This contributes to production costs.

THE DENESE TRANSLATION GUIDE TO SKIN-CARE INGREDIENTS

Here are some of the ingredients often found on skin-care product labels. I've put a star ☆ next to those that are especially useful and a flag ↶ next to those you should be careful about. Remember: comedogenic means the product is likely to cause clogged pores and possibly acne breakouts; noncomedogenic means the product has been designed not to cause clogged pores.

↶ **Acetylated lanolin alcohol** an ingredient to avoid. In general, lanolin is highly comedogenic and can lead to whiteheads and blackheads. It is usually used as a moisturizer. It is an alcohol that is not drying.

☆ **Alcohol SD-40** a high-grade purified cosmetics alcohol. It evaporates instantly, so it is used as a vehicle to transport important ingredients to the skin's surface. It then leaves the substance behind. It is less drying than ethyl alcohol.

☆ **Algae/Seaweed Extract** contains antioxidant properties. Normally used as an emollient that restores moisture content to skin.

☆ **Allantoin** a botanical extract believed to be calming for skin irritation.

☆ **Alpha-hydroxy acids or fruit acids** include many different substances such as citric acid (citrus fruits), glycolic acid (sugarcane), lactic acid (milk), and the less common malic acid (apples) and tartaric acid (wine). Helps exfoliate the top layers of the epidermis and helps to enable the penetration of other ingredients. Also improves skin moisture content. Key ingredients in anti-aging and skin bleaching products. They can be irritating to the skin; however, they do not cause the skin to age faster; if anything, the opposite is the case. AHAs increase sun sensitivity due to their exfoliant action.

☆ **Alphalipoic acid** an antioxidant that has been shown to penetrate the skin because it is both water- and fat-soluble. This means that it can be present in both the inside and the outside of the cell. It is also anti-inflammatory, which may help to reduce puffiness and redness in the skin.

☆ **Ascorbyl palmitate** a form of vitamin C. Less effective for building collagen, but more stable.

☆ **Benzoyl peroxide** an antibacterial agent that kills the germ responsible for acne flare-ups. Can be drying and/or irritating. Available in both prescription and over-the-counter forms, with percentages ranging from 2 to 10 percent solutions.

☆ **Beta-hydroxy acid** also known as salicylic acid. Used for exfoliation of dry skin and for acne therapy. Legal limit is only 2 percent strength in skin-care preparations.

☆ **Caffeine** alleviates under-eye puffiness and drains fluids from cellulite-ridden areas of the body.

☞ **Camphor** a cooling agent, alleviates itching and irritation, dries the skin.

☆ **Caviar extract** fish eggs are high in mineral and vitamin content (B_1, B_2, B_6, as well as A, E, and D). Promoted as useful for improving the appearance of maturing skin.

☆ **Ceramides** lipids (fats) that are almost identical in structure to human skin lipids. They are key in re-creating the all-important skin lipid barrier that protects the skin from drying out, and they are especially important to use in dry desert climates, in cold weather, or in dry indoor heat.

☆ **Cetyl alcohol** a lubricant that also emulsifies oil and water formulations. It's nonirritating, nondrying, and won't provoke acne.

☆ **Collagen** the main supporting fiber within the dermis. Gives strength and provides structure to skin. You cannot replace lost collagen by applying it to your skin, as it is incapable of penetration due to its large size. Topical collagen is able to moisturize and hydrate by holding many times its own weight in water.

☆ **Cyclic acid** a new term for hyaluronic acid, a strong hydrating complex that can hold a thousand times the water in skin.

☆ **Cyclomethicone** a form of silicone that gives products a smooth texture without blocking pores. Noncomedogenic.

☆ **Dimethicone** another form of silicone. Gives slip and glide to products. Has been used in some scar therapies. Noncomedogenic.

EDTA a preservative. Can cause contact dermatitis in sensitive skin.

☆ **Elastin** a fiber within the dermis similar to collagen. When inside the skin, it gives support and resilience to the skin. In topical products it cannot penetrate the skin due to its large size, but it is great for protecting against moisture loss.

☞ **Ethyl alcohol (aka rubbing alcohol or ethanol)** has an antibacterial function, but it is a bad irritant and very drying to the skin.

☆ **Glycerin** found in most products. Hydrates and provides a skin barrier. Allows topical agents to go on very smoothly. Can clog pores when present in high concentrations.

☆ **Glycine** an amino acid vital to collagen composition and production.

☆ **Glycolic acid** an alpha-hydroxy acid helpful for acne-prone skin. Resolves dry skin conditions. Used in chemical peels, as well as to help reduce the appearance of pores and wrinkles. Exfoliates excess flaking or crusty skin.

Glycol stearate a thickening agent that helps give products a luminescent or opalescent appearance.

Grapeseed extract a botanical extract shown to be an effective antioxidant.

☆ **Green tea extract** a powerful antioxidant.

☆ **Hyaluronic acid** an excellent hydrating substance. Best used in serum form. It can leave skin feeling dry if you do not add some skin-identical lipids (ceramides) to seal it in.

☆ **Hydroquinone** skin pigment lightening agent. A maximum of 2 percent may be obtained over-the-counter; higher concentrations available by prescription (4 to 6 percent). Best used in combination with glycolic acid or retinol for skin-fading purposes.

Isopropyl alcohol contains antibacterial properties, but can be drying to the skin, especially in high concentrations.

Isopropyl isostearate an emollient.

Isopropyl palmitate a moisturizing emollient. It has no allergic potential, although it is derived from palm and/or coconut oils. Comedogenic in nature.

☆ **Kaolin** used in oil-absorbing powders and masques; highly absorbent.

☆ **Kojic acid** a skin lightener.

☆ **Lactic acid** an alpha-hydroxy acid used in dermatology to hydrate and smooth dry, flaking skin. May occasionally be used in higher concentrations (above 12 percent) as a chemical peel.

☞ **Lanolin** an emollient and moisturizer. Obtained from sheep. Can cause allergic reactions. Rarely used in good-grade skin-care preparations anymore. Very comedogenic.

☆ **L-ascorbic acid (aka vitamin C)** used as an antioxidant in its l-ascorbic acid form, can have a skin-lightening effect in certain preparations. It's an essential component in building collagen.

☆ **Lecithin** a water-attracting agent used in products to help hydrate and improve the texture of the skin and to ease the spread of other ingredients onto the skin.

☆ **Licorice extract** skin lightener. More potent than kojic acid or vitamin C for this function.

☆ **Linoleic acid (aka vitamin F)** used to create emulsions. See the vitamins table earlier in this chapter.

☆ **Lysine** an amino acid and skin conditioner.

☞ **Octyl methoxycinnamate** an FDA–approved chemical sunscreen. Has contact dermatitis potential in some individuals.

☆ **Oxybenzone** an FDA–approved UVA–absorbing chemical sunscreen ingredient.

☞ **PABA (para–aminobenzoic acid)** UVB absorber used in sunscreens during the 1970s. Became a frequent cause of contact dermatitis; therefore it is now out of favor.

☆ **Panthenol** a B vitamin (B_5). Works as a humectant (holds water in the skin). May promote healing.

Parabens preservatives that are deemed safe and unlikely to irritate the skin. Widely used for cosmetics. Various forms will be listed with the ingredient (e.g., methylparaben, propylparaben, butylparaben).

☞ **Petrolatum** a heavy bland base, most commonly known for its use in Vaseline. Good for lips but not for other skin. It is occlusive and can cause plugging of the pores and acne in prone individuals. Strongly comedogenic.

Polybutene helps make liquids texturally viscous.

Polyhydroxy acid (PHA) derived from the buds of fruit trees. Claims to be gentler, yet as effective as AHAs. Still debatable.

☆ **Proline** an amino acid vital to the composition and production of collagen.

☆ **Resveratrol** an antioxidant that supports and protects collagen.

☆ **Retinol** a derivative of vitamin A. Fat-soluble. Depending on concentration, estimated to be approximately ten times less effective than tretinoin.

☆ **Retinyl palmitate (aka vitamin A palmitate)** considered a more stable alternative to retinol for normalizing the skin's texture and helping smooth out fine lines. It's the ester of retinol combined with palmitic acid and thought to be less irritating than retinol.

☆ **Retinyl palmitate polypeptide** a water-soluble formulation of vitamin A.

☆ **Rose hips** a botanical extract of rose petals found to have high concentrations of vitamin C.

☆ **Salicylic acid** classified as a BHA (beta-hydroxy acid). Medically used as an exfoliant and debriding agent. Cosmetically used in some chemical peels and to reduce oiliness, acne, and the appearance of fine lines.

Silicone shields the skin and creates a sheen. Thought to be helpful in reducing the appearance of some scars. Noncomedogenic.

Silk powder incorporated into cosmetics powders to help absorb skin moisture and oils.

☆ **Silk proteins** prevents dehydration. Commonly found in eye rejuvenation creams.

☆ **Sodium hyaluronate** related to hyaluronic acid (salt form). Works to moisturize the skin; can hold more than a thousand times its own weight in water.

Sodium laurel sulfate found in most cleansers and soaps. Acts as a surfactant. Offers good foaming qualities. A known skin irritant, but contrary to popular myths, does not cause cancer.

Sulfur helps kill normal bacteria on the skin, improving acne, seborrhea, and psoriasis conditions. Typically found in soaps, shampoos, and some topical acne medications.

☆ **Titanium dioxide** a UV blocker. Helps block both UVA and UVB wavelengths of light.

☆ **Tyrosine** an amino acid that in in-vitro studies stimulates fibroblasts to make more collagen when paired with ascorbic acid. Plays a role in melanin formation.

Wax provides moisture as well as a barrier function. Allows for oil and water blending (emulsion).

☆ **Witch hazel** botanical with astringent properties. Helps remove excess surface skin oils.

Xanthan gum an agent used to thicken the ingredients in many products.

☆ **Zinc oxide** the broadest-spectrum UVA/UBA sunscreen available today. The only drawback is its pasty white color. More advanced products reduce the particles into a micronized form for easier application and penetration.

NEWLY EMERGING INGREDIENTS IN SKIN CARE

Here is the cutting edge in the science of beauty. It may be difficult for you to find products that contain some of these powerful anti-aging chemicals, but keep your eyes open. They are worth looking for in the world of cosmeceuticals.

• *Bioactive amino acid peptides.* These molecular structures (they can be tripeptides [three peptides joined together], tetrapeptides [four], pentaptides [five], or hexapeptides [six]) have the great advantage of being small enough to penetrate the skin. In various in-vitro studies they have been able to turn on cellular machinery to significantly increase collagen and elastin production and to protect from premature collagen destruction in the skin. With each passing month, better and more effective ones appear on the raw-ingredients market.

Not all peptides are created equal; some are more effective than others. One pentapeptide, marketed as Matrixyl, an ingredient found in many cosmetics, is composed of a combination of amino acids that mimics nature's tissue-regenerating processes by signaling the cells of the dermis to synthesize proteins. Two teams of investigators have reported that it is as effective as retinol in improving the effects of skin aging, but without the side effects often associated with retinol.

You might think that major cosmetics houses would jump at the opportunity presented by these powerful peptides, but the companies are slow to respond and, as I'm sure you can guess, they tend to use these exceedingly expensive ingredients only in very small amounts.

• *Carnosine.* Recent research identifies this small molecule, composed of amino acids, as the most promising broad-spectrum shield against nearly all of the physiological processes that destroy protein and make us age, such as glycation and protein carbonylation. To a large extent, it's protein destruction that's responsible for skin aging. A vast number of scientific studies show that carnosine protects protein and, to some extent, can reverse the damage.

In my opinion, carnosine may bring about some revolutionary changes in skin care, but it is in very few products on the market. I have a serum with carnosine, called Growth Factor Serum, but I would be hard-pressed to name another product that contains it. However, this may soon change.

• *Copper peptides.* Copper, an essential nutrient for the skin, has long been used in medicine to speed the healing of burns. In clinical studies, copper peptides promote tissue building, help heal collagen and elastin damage, and improve the appearance of fine lines and wrinkles. ProCyte is the company that holds the patent for the most effective skin delivery method for copper peptides. Ingredients to look for are prexatide copper acetate, copper tripeptide-1, alanine/histadine, or lysine ploypeptide-copper HCl, all of which can be found in a line of products under the brand-name Neova.

• *Epidermal growth factor (EPF).* This healing agent is derived from recombinant DNA/RNA, and in clinical as well as in in-vitro studies it has been shown to increase circulation, synthesis of protein, fibroblast production, and accumulation of collagen. It may contribute to improvement in skin texture, the appearance of wrinkle depth, and skin elasticity. There are a few serums that boast epidermal and other dermal growth factors among their ingredients. Two examples are: Transformé Epidermal Growth Factor and Skin Therapy EGF Cream.

An ingredient marketed as Nouricel-MD is rich in human growth factors, amino acids, soluble collagen, antioxidants, and matrix proteins, and is found in a 93.2 percent concentration in a product called TNS Recovery Complex. While it sounds promising, it is still not the Holy Grail, so please look for genuine changes in your skin. If you don't see any in a few weeks, find a new product that does more for

THE JURY IS STILL OUT

For the sake of completeness, here are a few other products and ingredients on the market that offer unique promises you may need further guidelines to interpret.

BOSWELLIC ACIDS. These are proinflammatory enzymes that can stimulate collagen. The standardized extract that contains these enzymes is called boswellin, a new ingredient with great, sudden repute. But to put it in perspective, although proinflammatory enzymes are very important, they are a relatively small piece of the puzzle of aging. L'Oréal's Wrinkle De-Crease contains boswellox, a phyto-complex combining boswellic acid and manganese. This product claims to reduce the appearance of expression lines and wrinkles within three weeks. My advice is to try it and see if it works for you, but don't settle for anything less than genuine changes in your skin before you commit yourself to the product.

BOTOX ALTERNATIVES After these antiwrinkle injections hit the market, the cosmetics industry rolled out an array of active ingredients that are said to mimic the action of Botox. In general, these products are minimally effective in comparison to the injections, so keep your eyes open and do not settle. The most popular of these products are:

- Avotox, which contains 10 percent acetyl hexapeptide-3 (Argireline), works through a unique mechanism to relax facial tension to a very minimal degree, leading to a reduction in the appearance of superficial lines and wrinkles with regular use.

- Bioque Serum XL, which contains 15 percent acetyl hexapeptide-3.

- StriVectin SD, which contains Striadril Complex, consisting of palmitoyl pentapeptide 3, palmitoyl oligo-peptide, and numerous botanical extracts. Strictly speaking, this product does not fall in the category of skin relaxers, even though it markets itself as such. Its effect is based on the collagen-stimulating effects of amino acid peptides.

In my opinion, the effectiveness of these products is very minimal compared to Botox injections.

ESTROGEN, PROGESTERONE, TESTOSTERONE. Hormonal decline is an intrinsic factor in skin aging, but topical, nonprescription creams are not allowed, by law, to contain enough of these hormones to make a difference in the structure of the skin. However, if you need hormone replacement anyway, talk to your doctor. It can be worthwhile to apply your hormone replacement directly on the face, upon your doctor's approval. It will improve your estrogen levels, and at the same time it may improve your skin thickness. The idea of improving skin thickness by the direct application of estriol, a safe, natural estrogen, is based on a scientific study. But the level of estriol required here is prescription-strength only, so you must consult your doctor if you wish to try this treatment.

you. The problem with pure epidermal growth factor, at the moment, is the price. The last time I priced it, one gram (about the size of a pinch of salt) of epidermal growth factor from France was $100,000, and I was told that was a very good price.

Fortunately, studies show that serums rich is bioamino peptides can favorably compete with the effectiveness of TNS Recovery Complex, so they are an excellent alternative until the price of EPF comes down.

DR. DENESE'S GUIDE TO SPA SERVICES

In recent years, spas and salons have been offering a vast array of beauty treatments. Just like at the cosmetics counter, it's up to you, the savvy consumer, to figure out what kind of service and experience you want, and find the place and treatment that suit you best.

Many spas and salons are expensive; while you're having your back rubbed you may also be having your wallet massaged. But if you can afford it, the physical benefits of spa treatments can do wonders for your psyche. We all deserve a little pampering and relief from the stresses of this world. Being spoiled by relaxing facials, wrapped in aromatic mud and seaweed, massaged into Zen-like bliss by warm and firm professional hands can elevate your spirit for a few hours. The question is, how do you hold on to the state of relaxation? It is worth it if it makes you feel good and you know what you are getting. Because, let me tell you, you are not getting much—not to keep, anyway. The benefits of salon and spa treatments, in my opinion, are fleeting.

There are several types of facilities to choose from:

• Destination and resort spas, such as Canyon Ranch, that have a staff of physicians, psychologists, nutritionists, and physical therapists and offer so many exercise classes, lectures, and services that it appears overwhelming at first. Do not be intimidated by them. Most importantly, do not feel left out if you cannot afford to stay there for a week or two, because you are not missing out on the Fountain of Youth. Take it from me, a scientist: there is a lot of fluff there to justify the expense, but none of these places hold the key to eternal youth. They do not give you any more than a nice vacation, although you may lose a little weight as a benefit of the consistent exercise and good diet. If you can maintain what you learn about diet and exercise and continue to practice a healthy lifestyle, it's worth the price of admission.

• Day spas and salons that provide professionally administered massages, facials, and body treatments in a quiet, serene atmosphere. It feels great while it lasts; the problem is that the benefits of plumped-up lines do not last beyond a day or two. Let's take a quick look at the treatments available:

Body polishing and exfoliating body scrubs. These provide nothing that you can't replicate at home with readily available salt scrubs and other body products.

Cellulite-reducing spa treatments. I don't know a woman over thirty who does not think she has cellulite. Cellulite is fibrous tissue that develops inside the subcutaneous fat layer. The fibrous tissue articulates the fat into pockets, so from the outside the fat looks dimpled. It is much like a down quilt, the way the fat is sorted into pockets and separated by fibrous walls. This down quilt lies over the muscles, so even if you are toned, it may not show from beneath the fibrous fat (cellulite) layer. Often the cellulite layer holds water, which makes it appear even more dimpled. If you drain the water, the appearance of cellulite will diminish. Seaweed and cellulite wraps are based on this principle: you lose water and appear to lose size after a treatment. The problem is that it is strictly temporary. Some unscrupulous cellulite-reducing centers may claim to provide treatment that breaks down the fibrous tissue that makes cellulite. This is where you have to draw the line. It is impossible to break down fibrous tissue from the outside. These claims are banking on the fact that few people know what a surgeon knows: that the fibers that hold cellulite are so strong, they can't be broken by hands; they have to be cut. So how could a wrap or a cellulite massage, however sophisticated, break down the fibers under the skin?

Endermology. This is a suctioning treatment that uses a sophisticated vacuum device to reduce the look of cellulite. It can improve lymphatic circulation and effectively drain cellulitic areas, but it is not a permanent solution for cellulite, although better than most.

Lymphatic massage. This can be very pleasant and more useful than most spa treatments, if delivered properly. It is a gentle massage that is intended to return the lymphatic fluid into the blood circulation. As we grow older, lymphatic circulation can get sluggish, so there is validity to a treatment that can effectively encourage lymphatic return.

Herbal body wraps and seaweed detoxifying treatments. Body wraps can make you lose water effectively from the tissue that is wrapped. It is possible that your legs may appear to be thinner after the wrap, but the magic does not last long. You may gain the water back promptly.

• Alternative medicine spas, offering Ayurveda treatments and other cross-cultural beauty and health therapies. These facilities claim to reverse the aging process by arresting the degeneration of the body cells and improving the immune system. Here's my opinion: I wish it were so easy. I find these claims vastly exaggerated and scientifically naive. I do not think that these processes are harmful, they may even be of some benefit, but one should not overstate the benefits without reliable scientific studies to back the claims.

• Medical spas. These are the places that will actually have more than a fleeting impact on your looks. They are run by doctors with expertise in cosmetic dermatology, and they offer a full range of medical care, including Botox injections and wrinkle filler injections; skin resurfacing with light, medium, and deep laser peels and chemical peels; removal of tattoos and unwanted hair; and treatment of telangiectasia ("broken" capillaries). These are skills that can only be learned the hard way—via the solid foundation that only a medical training can provide.

Please, do not let a nonmedical person inject anything in you (it is against the law, anyway) or use a laser (hair removal, vein removal) on you without direct, on-site medical supervision. Always ask if there is a doctor in the house before your treatment starts. Insist that the doctor personally check the laser settings before your laser treatment begins. Once the laser starts flashing and possibly burning your skin, it will be too late. I have seen too many cases of unprofessional laser hair removal from the face, and met too many victims who ended up with permanent marks.

So there you have it. Go out shopping: visit some spas and doctors' offices. Come back prettier than when you left and tell us what you have learned.

CHAPTER ELEVEN

ASK DR. DENESE

1. I have marionette lines on my face. I'm thinking about getting a filler to deal with them. How do I know which filler to ask for?

There are so many cosmetic fillers on the market today and the field develops so rapidly that it can get a bit confusing. So let us review some of the newest additions to the family.

As you know, the history of cosmetic fillers began with bovine (cow) collagen more than twenty years ago. Bovine collagen is rarely used these days because it is short-lived (a few weeks) and there is a very high potential for allergic reactions.

Recently the FDA approved a bioengineered human collagen that consists of collagen originally derived from human cells. While this bioengineered human collagen does not pose the same allergy risk as traditional bovine collagen, the results are still very short-lived (two to three months) compared to other fillers.

Another soft-tissue filler that received FDA approval recently is a nonanimal-derived hyaluronic acid under the trade name of Restyline (or Peryline, a similar substance still awaiting approval at the time of this book's printing). Hyaluronic acid is a naturally occurring component of the skin. Compared to collagen, hyaluronic acid works better in improving nasolabial folds and marionette lines. The results last longer (four to six months), there is no allergy risk, and there is no risk of transmitting animalborne diseases. It has been used in Canada, Europe, and Australia with great success and is regarded by many doctors as perhaps one of the most superior fillers that currently exists.

For patients who want longer-lasting results, there is a new filler known by the trade name Radiance. This new scientific filler contains beads of hydroxyapatite, a substance normally used to replace missing bone.

For patients looking for permanent wrinkle fillers, one of the new injectables currently awaiting FDA approval in the United States is polymethylmethacrylate. This is made from a mixture of micronized plastic spheres and bovine collagen. Polymethylmethacrylate has been shown to work well for moderate to deep wrinkles and scars, but it is not recommended for lips. The results of polymethylmethacrylate are permanent, so it is extremely important that you go to a dermatologist or surgeon who is experienced in the procedure.

My suggestion is to start with a nonpermanent hyaluronic acid-based injection and see how you like the effect. Afterward you can move on to a more permanent filler.

2. How should I decide if I need a face-lift and if it will help me?

First, look into the mirror. The most important indication for surgical intervention is in the jawline and the neck. If you see jowls and if that troubles you, you have to face the fact that no topical treatments can make the situation better.

You can tell what a face-lift would look like by lifting the skin by the temples. Push against your temples and move your fingers upward. Don't pull your face backward. That will give you the undesirable windswept, old face-lift look. Pulling the skin upward will give you a truer understanding. This is how a well-done modern mini face-lift should look: subtle. All of your features should be essentially unchanged, yet the face looks about ten years younger.

3. What is the difference between a scrub and a microdermabrasion cream?

Scrubs in general have coarser granules. They're usually based on some natural product such as apricot shells or walnut shells. Microdermabrasion creams use very fine particles, most often aluminum oxide or talc, to give a micropolish to the skin. Coarse particles scratch the skin, and that's not what you want. What you want is to give a very even and defined micropolish to the skin to remove old dead skin cells and stimulate cellular turnover and the cells' own machinery for collagen regeneration.

4. There are a lot of pore strips on the market now. You stick them on your nose or chin and then peel them off after a few minutes; they supposedly pull dirt and blackheads out of pores. Do they really work, and are they a good idea?

This would be a very good idea if it worked, but unfortunately the package usually promises more than it can deliver. The dirt is much deeper in the pores and really can't be accessed by these simple means. Some of the superficial dirt particles will certainly come off, but the ones we really care about—the deep-seeded, pore-clogging particles— I do not think will come out with pore strips.

5. How effective are the over-the-counter creams that claim to destroy fat deposits and thereby prevent cellulite and the "cottage cheese" look on legs and thighs?

I wish it were that easy. A cream that can reduce cellulite and fat deposits—that would be a miracle! Unfortunately, such a cream does not exist, because it's nearly impossible to get rid of fat deposits from under the skin by applying a topical product. The effect of such a cream, if any, is minimal and is based on draining fluid from the area rather than attacking fat or the cellulitic structure. A cream can drain fluid, but fluid will come back promptly in a few days.

6. In the winter, my legs become extremely dry, scaly, and itchy. On occasion I've been driven to scratch them so much they've bled. And no amount of moisturizing lotion seems to alleviate the problem. What do you suggest?

The most important thing you can do to correct this problem is to exfoliate the skin. Part of the reason that you are unable to put moisture back into the skin is that there is so much accumulated dead old skin that moisture can't penetrate properly. Exfoliation will allow the moisturizer you put on to access your skin much more successfully. You can do mechanical scrubbing with a loofah or sponge; use a microdermabrasion cream; or better yet, I'd recommend glycolic acid peel pads. You can use your facial pads if you have none other; however, there are larger-size glycolic acid peel pads intended for the body currently on the market. They are a bit stronger than the facial pads, so they work even better on coarser body skin. I prefer glycolic acid–based exfoliation to a loofah because it does not scratch dry, fragile skin and delivers a more uniform exfoliation.

7. Are loofahs and dry body brushes a good way to remove dead skin cells from my arms, legs, torso, and back?

Yes, certainly there's no harm in using loofahs or body brushes; they do exfoliate. But I think we need something a bit more sophisticated. Loofahs and body brushes are too coarse for the skin. You wind up overscratching certain parts and not polishing other parts at all. Whatever the loofah doesn't reach does not get exfoliated. I think you'd be better served with a strong, large-size glycolic acid peel pad. That will exfoliate the skin more uniformly.

8. I've read that facial exercises will help tone the muscles just as regular exercise tones the rest of the body. I've also heard that facial massage and pinching the underlying muscle and tissue will work the muscles and keep them from becoming flaccid and droopy, thus slowing down the onset of wrinkles. Is there any truth to this?

This is not an easy question to answer. First, pinching the muscles has nothing to do with wrinkling or drooping whatsoever, so we can eliminate that part of the question right away. Now, facial exercises may sound like a good idea, but think about it: all your wrinkles come about as a result of facial exercises. The wrinkles around the eyes come about from smiling and moving the muscles underneath. The lines around the mouth emerge after moving the lips (talking, smiling, eating, etc.) for many years. So why would moving these muscles even more than they already do decrease the amount of lines on your face?

As you know, facial muscles originate on the bone and attach directly to the skin. So every time you move the skin, you pull the muscle with it, generating more and more lines. That's why I'm not sure that facial exercise will get you the results you are looking for, since moving the muscles is what causes lines in the first place. There is a certain electrical machine that stimulates deeper muscles under the skin of the face. I've seen good results from it. But exercising the muscles on your own will not get you very far.

9. Is getting a superficial peel in your mid-twenties a good idea? Or is it better to wait until at least the thirties, when some of the aging signs are more prominent?

If you have absolutely flawless skin, then getting superficial peels is truly a waste. On the other hand, if you have any evidence of clogged pores, bumpiness under the skin, or acne, then superficial peels are definitely a very good idea. In fact, combining the superficial peel with aggressive anti-acne and exfoliating treatments is a very successful method for treating any of these problems.

10. You say that sun damages skin, but what about tanning booths? Are they less damaging?

The tanning booths are actually nearly as damaging as the sun itself, so please, stay away.

11. Is the dry heat of a sauna or the humid heat of a steam room good for my skin?

They are certainly good for your health, but don't expect anti-aging benefits. The sauna and steam room promote circulation, a very important and positive effect on the body.

12. Can vitamins and nutrition prevent acne?

We would love to think so, but unfortunately there is really no scientific evidence to support the connection. There are some vitamins (particularly vitamins A, B_5, B_6, and E) that can assist in your efforts to fight acne, but there's truly no proven, clear-cut relationship. There is some evidence that eating a sugar-laden or very fatty diet can possibly induce acne outbreaks. But even there, the relationship is very weak.

13. Why am I getting acne on my back, and what can I do about it?

Acne on the back is a very prevalent problem, so don't feel alone. The first part of your question is the more important one from the perspective of prevention.

If you suddenly develop acne on your back, chances are high that it's environmentally induced. The following are possibilities for why you are breaking out on the back: summer heat, being overheated under heavy covers at night during the winter, noncotton sheets that touch your sweaty back at night, heavy exercise with associated sweating, fabrics that do not allow the skin to air (heavy winter fabrics or tight polyester T-shirts in the summer), and not reaching your back to give it a good scrub during showers. Then there's always stress and hormonal changes, just to name two.

What can you do about it? AHA/BHA peels on your back work wonders to unclog pores and exfoliate the skin to prevent clogging and accumulation of oily plugs under the skin. You can have it done professionally at great expense of both time and money, or use professional-grade glycolic and salicylic acid acne peel pads at home, at your leisure, for pennies a day. If these treatments fail, go for professional versions of these peels and microdermabrasion treatments.

14. Someone told me I should use a different set of products for the summer than the winter. Were they just trying to sell me more products?

The season matters a great deal. Winter skin care needs to emphasize the skin barrier function. Cold winter air is harsh and has very low humidity. To top it off, dry indoor heat also has very low humidity, so your skin does not get a break in the winter, indoors or out. Low humidity, dry heat, and cold air dry the skin. The most important adjustment you have to make during the winter is to increase your use of products that have ceramides and essential fatty acids to fortify the skin lipid barrier. Elizabeth Arden has a ceramide serum called Bye-Lines Anti-Aging Serum that can serve this function well. The signature product in my line, HydroShield Serum, is highly effective.

There are some excellent creams on the market (from inexpensive to very expensive) that promote barrier function well, such as:

- Elizabeth Arden Ceramide Plump Perfect Moisture Cream SPF30

- RoC Retinol Actif Pur Anti-Wrinkle Moisturizing Treatment Day/Night

- L'Oréal Revitalift Anti-Wrinkle and Firming Night Cream

- Estée Lauder Resilience Lift Eye Cream

- Clarins Multi-Active Jour-Line Prevention Day Cream

- Clarins Multi Active Nuit-Line-Prevention Lotion

- Clarins Extra Firming Day/Night Cream

- Clinique Repairwear Intensive Night Cream

- Lancôme Primordiale Optimum Night Cream

- NeoStrata Bio-Hydrating Cream

For the summer, continue with exfoliation and the skin-stimulating phase of skin care, but lighten up on night creams.

15. Is there any validity to the lip plumper creams?

You are the best judge of that. There is a whole array of lip plumpers on the market. Try a few and see how they work for you. Lip plumpers should give your lips a temporary boost. The plumping effect should be visible and obvious; otherwise it is not a good plumper. The plumping effect comes about by inducing extra circulation in the lips, mostly via temporarily irritating the skin. The irritation causes no harm. However, after stretching or irritating the mucous membrane, your lips will be more dry than before. It is important to follow up with a good, occlusive lip balm to allow the lips to heal themselves. Some products claim to help facilitate the building of collagen in the lips with amino peptide ingredients. It is possible, but you need high percentages of the active ingredients, so look for fairly expensive products from a reputable, established company.

16. What is the best way to find a dermatologist in my area? Is there a professional organization for dermatologists?

The organization is called American Dermatology Association (ADA). It is very prominent and can be easily accessed on the Internet. They have rosters of dermatologists in your area. If you are looking for a new dermatologist, the best way to find out if a particular doctor is a good one is word of mouth—it's a very powerful tool. Also, look for advertisements in upscale local leisure magazines. Dermatologists who have prominent, cosmetically oriented practices are the only ones who can afford the advertising. And they usually provide very good service. Look for a breadth of services. The more comprehensive a doctor's offerings, the better equipped he or she is to handle your problem. Try to stay away from dermatologists who do only one or two procedures.

GLOSSARY

Accutane An extremely aggressive tretinoin-based product used as a last resort to heal cystic acne. It is highly effective, but it can cause severe birth defects in pregnant women. In very rare cases it can even cause depression.

Acetyl-l-carnitine An antioxidant that promotes the health and rejuvenation of mitochondrial and membrane functions, combating the aging process.

Alpha-hydroxy acids (AHA) A supercategory of anti-inflammatory, exfoliating acids (derived from fruit, milk, etc.) that includes glycolic, lactic, malic, and fruit acids.

Alphalipoic acid An important anti-aging antioxidant.

Amino acids Biochemical building blocks. They form long chemical chains called proteins and shorter chains called peptides.

Androgen hormones Any of the steroid hormones that develop and maintain masculine characteristics. Testosterone is one such hormone. A surge of these hormones in puberty or menopause often causes cystic acne by increasing the production of sebum.

Angulation The angling or "cornering" of the skin on the neck.

Antioxidants Chemicals that prevent and reverse the production of highly reactive free radicals, which can readily damage other molecules. The presence of antioxidants can "mop up" free radicals before they damage essential molecules.

Arbutin A skin-fading chemical.

Argireline An amino acid that relaxes and smoothes wrinkles. A topical alternative to Botox.

Beta-hydroxy acids (BHA) A group of exfoliating acids. The major one is salicylic acid.

Botox Botulinum toxin. A muscle relaxant that, when injected directly into the muscles of the skin, can temporarily smooth wrinkle lines.

Botswella An amino acid that relaxes and smoothes wrinkles. A topical alternative to Botox.

Capillaries The smallest of the body's blood vessels. Capillaries have walls so thin that oxygen and glucose can pass through them and enter the cells, and waste products such as carbon dioxide can pass back into the blood to be taken out of the body.

Carnosine An antioxidant within muscle tissue. It is composed of two amino acids joined by a peptide bond. An important ingredient in a skin-stimulating serum, it revitalizes and regenerates skin fibroblasts.

Cellular turnover The rate at which cells die and are replaced by new ones.

Ceramide A lipid (fat) identical in composition to the skin's natural lipid molecules. An effective ingredient in lipid-based moisturizing serums.

Chemical peel The removal of layers of the skin via chemical means (i.e., using acids to slough off cells).

Collagen The main protein in the connective tissues of the body. It is responsible for skin elasticity, and its degradation leads to wrinkles that accompany aging.

Comedones These occur when excess sebaceous oil and dead skin cells combine to clog the hair follicle inside a pore. When a comedone breaks through the skin, it becomes a whitehead, blackhead, or pimple.

Cortisol A hormone that promotes aging by causing muscle breakdown, uncontrollable midsection weight gain, and thinning of the skin.

Cystic acne Inflamed, red pustular acne with a deep nodular base. It is the most severe form of acne and usually has a hormonal component—that is, it's often caused by a sudden surge of androgen hormones.

Deep peel The deepest, most dramatic peel, which reaches far into the dermal skin layer to regenerate collagen. It can be chemical or mechanical, but laser peels offer the most control. Involves anesthesia and weeks, even months of recovery time, since the skin is literally burned off.

Dermabrasion A procedure that uses a machine resembling a dentist's drill, which sands or buffs the top (dead) layer of skin, forcing collagen production and stimulating skin thickness. Aggressive use of sun block is required after the procedure, and the skin is sensitive and often swollen.

Dermis The layer of skin underneath the epidermis. It contains a number of structures including blood vessels, nerves, hair follicles, smooth muscles, glands, and lymphatic tissue. It is made up of dense collagen and other fibers.

EFA Essential fatty acids (such as linoleic acid) present in lipid-based serums that build up and moisturize the skin.

Enzymatic peel A peel that uses enzymes to "eat away" at skin layers as a method of exfoliation.

Enzymes Proteins that act as catalysts. They speed up the rate at which biochemical reactions proceed but don't alter the direction or nature of the reaction.

Epidermis The outermost layer of the skin. It contains no blood vessels and is nourished by diffusion from the dermis.

Erbium laser New laser technology that causes less heating and burning of tissues than other lasers used in skin resurfacing. In comparison to older, more conventional methods, it is less painful and has a shorter healing time.

Estrogen The main sex hormone that regulates female reproductive processes and creates feminine secondary sexual characteristics. Depletion in estrogen can lead to thinning skin, loss of elasticity, and increasing lines.

Exfoliation The process of sloughing off dead skin cells from the epidermis.

FDA (Food and Drug Administration) A branch of the U.S. federal government's Department of Health and Human Services. It is responsible for promoting and protecting the public health by ensuring that safe and healthy products get on the market and banning dangerous ones from importation and sale.

Fibroblasts Cells that make up the structural fibers of connective tissue (i.e., collagen).

Free radicals Uncharged atomic particles with unpaired electrons. These molecules are unstable and therefore highly reactive. They oxidize with the more stable chemicals of the body and compromise cellular functioning to promote aging. Antioxidants play a key role in the defense against free radicals.

Frequency-based laser rejuvenation A type of laser treatment that uses radio-frequency waves to stimulate cellular turnover.

Fruit acid A water-soluble antioxidant derived from various fruits (straw-berries, tomatoes, apples, etc.) containing vitamin C. It aids in the production of collagen.

Glucagon The natural antidote to insulin. It is a hormone that speeds up metabolism and reverses the aging effects of glycation. It cannot do so while high insulin levels are present, so it is important to keep the body's blood sugar levels down to allow glucagon to do its work.

Glycation The process whereby excess sugar molecules link and compro-mise cellular particles (such as DNA and other proteins), causing a break-down of functions and aging. Combated by keeping blood sugar levels low.

Glycolic acid An alpha-hydroxy acid. It is an exfoliant and a collagen stim-ulant that is most effective when used in no less than 8 to 10 percent strength solution. When used as a peel, it must be neutralized to keep it from peeling deeper than intended. Usually used in combination with salicylic acid.

Green makeup Covers up redness and irritation of the skin that can occur as a result of rosacea, telangiectasia, medium or deep peels, and any other skin-reddening condition.

Halogen light A light source with a more efficient, longer-lasting filament than regular lightbulbs.

Human growth hormone (HGH) Sometimes called the master hormone of youth. HGH is secreted at night by the pituitary gland and is responsible for helping the body grow, repair itself, and maintain proper functioning. HGH injections help to increase metabolism, improve brain performance, re-pair all of the body's tissues, and generally improve well-being.

Hyaluronic acid A peptide in skin-stimulating serums that also seals mois-ture in the skin. In addition, it is used as an injectable filler to reduce wrinkles on the face.

Hydroquinone A drug that inhibits the manufacture of new pigment cells and can lighten dark spots and discolorations.

Hyperinsulinemia Chronically elevated insulin levels.

Injectible fillers Any of the variety of synthetic or natural substances that can be injected into the muscles of the face to reduce the look of lines and wrinkles.

Insulin The hormone responsible for maintaining a proper balance of blood sugar in the body. It has profound pro-aging qualities. The degeneration of insulin receptors causes increased glycation and hastens aging.

Laser peel A process that uses laser energy to burn off dead skin layers.

Linoleic acid A lipid identical in composition to the skin's natural lipid molecules. An effective ingredient in lipid-based moisturizing serums.

Lipids Fatty, waxy, or oily compounds that are characteristically insoluble in water but readily soluble in organic solvents. Lipids contain carbon, hydrogen, and oxygen.

Lipid-soluble Dissolves in fats.

Lipofuscin Toxic cellular material that accumulates and causes aging by compromising membrane functions.

Liposomes and liposomal delivery system Liposomes are highly complex, microscopic lipid (fatty) spheres that encapsulate water and other ingredients. They are round shells of phospholipids, the basic components of human cell walls. Enclosing an ingredient within a liposome entraps it and keeps it fresh. Liposome encapsulation also improves an ingredient's concentration and duration at the target site, which can triple or quadruple its effectiveness. Liposomal delivery can bring any chemical into the body effectively and precisely, with the maximum results.

Macrodermabrasion A procedure of mechanical exfoliation of the outer layers of skin using negative (vacuum) pressure. This old technology often employs abrasive aluminum oxide and tends to require a lengthy recovery time.

Marionette lines Wrinkle lines that run down from the corners of the mouth.

Mechanical peel A procedure that uses a microdermabrasion machine, which emits a fine spray of crystals, salt, or aluminum particles to polish away old skin cells.

Medium peel An exfoliation procedure that goes deep enough to affect both the epidermal and dermal skin layers. Can be done chemically, with light dermabrasion or with a laser. Administered under anesthesia and requires about a week of recovery time. It should only be administered by a medical doctor.

Melanin A pigment in the skin, hair, and eyes. Melanin protects the skin from damage by ultraviolet (UV) light and is the pigment produced in response to damage by the sun, causing skin to tan (to protect itself against further damage). In albino mammals, melanin is the pigment that is missing from their bodies.

Melanocytes Pigment cells that swarm into an area of recent acne inflammation and bring pigment to the skin, often leaving a persistent dark spot.

Melasma Large, amorphous, dark discolorations on the skin.

Microdermabrasion The removal of dead skin cells by exfoliating with a granular substance.

Mitochondria The power plant of cells, which, if compromised by any of the numerous aging factors, can break down, leading to cellular damage.

Nasolabial folds Embedded wrinkle lines that run from the nose to the mouth.

Nonablative lasers Lasers that heat the dermis without causing open wounds to the epidermis, thereby minimizing recovery time.

Noncomedogenic Products that do not clog hair follicles and, in turn, create comedones.

Obagi System Developed by Zein Obagi, a Middle Eastern doctor, this harsh mix of Retin A/hydroquinone successfully fades skin discolorations but causes extreme irritation and peeling for the first several weeks.

Pearline An injectable filler in the hyaluronic acid family currently on the market. Can remain in the face for up to one year.

Peels Chemical, mechanical, and laser procedures that remove layers of skin to various depths to promote skin thickness and rejuvenation.

Peptides Any of a class of molecules that make up chains of amino acids and form the building blocks of proteins.

Petrolatum A mineral oil. Found in traditional creams, it is ineffective and can cause clogged pores, since it does not have a molecular makeup identical to that of natural skin lipids.

pH balance Percentage of hydrogen balance. Refers to the balance of a product's acidity or alkalinity. Healthy skin is slightly acidic to ward off infections. To preserve pH balance, cosmetics products should be slightly acidic as well.

Phytosphyngosine An anti-inflammatory, nonsteroidal agent that decreases the inflammation and swelling of acne without thinning the skin.

Pores Openings in the skin that produce sebaceous oil, which lubricates and moisturizes the skin as well as acidifying it to maintain proper pH balance and protect it against bacteria. Pores enlarge to accommodate a higher output of sebaceous oil (usually during puberty or due to heightened sun exposure).

Porphyrins A chemical released by the skin bacteria *Propionobacterium acnes,* which causes acne.

Portculaca An amino acid that relaxes and smoothes wrinkles. A topical alternative to Botox.

Pregnenolone An antioxidant that supports mitochondrial functions.

Prolactin A hormone that increases with age and promotes weight gain.

Propionobacterium acnes Otherwise known as *P. acnes,* it is the bacteria that reside on the surface of the skin, and when they settle into clogged pores, cause acne.

Proteins The "machines" of the cell, proteins are made up of long chains of amino acids.

Pustules Elevated lesions on the skin that contain pus (the major component of acne).

Radio-frequency laser peel A laser procedure that stimulates the skin at a deeper level, bypassing the epidermis and minimizing recovery time.

RDA Recommended Dietary Allowance of a nutrient is the amount Americans are advised to consume daily by the Institute of Medicine of the American Academy of Arts and Sciences.

Restyline An FDA-approved hyaluronic filler used to fill facial lines and wrinkles.

Resveratrol An antioxidant in red grapes that combats the aging effects of cell oxidation by free radicals.

Retin A/Renova Types of tretinoin products often prescribed to cure acne-plagued skin.

Retinol The most potent form of vitamin A. A lipid-soluble vitamin found in medications such as Accutane, it reduces the secretion of oils from glands.

Rosacea A chronic and progressive skin disease that causes redness and swelling of the face. It sometimes includes acnelike pustules.

Salicylic acid An oil-soluble beta-hydroxy acid in aspirin and topical skin-care products. It is safe to use because it stops working two to three minutes after application.

Sebaceous glands In the hair follicles, these glands secrete sebum, an oily substance that keeps skin from drying out.

Sebum Semifluid secretions from sebaceous glands that collect in pores, causing blockages, irritation (which often leads to acne), and enlarged pores.

Serum A water-based product that is the best way to transfer collagen-building materials into the skin as part of the skin-stimulating phase. The main ingredient is water; other important ingredients are carnosine, resveratrol, bioactive oligopeptides, copper, vitamin C, and vitamin B complex.

Skin lipid barrier A layer of fat molecules under the skin's surface that keeps moisture in the skin. A breakdown of this layer of fats causes skin to be increasingly dry.

SPF Sun protection factor. SPF is essential to protect the skin from severe aging effects of sun exposure. SPF 15 is the least that should be applied, but SPF 30 is recommended.

Spironolactone A steroid used medically as a diuretic that prevents excessive oil production by blocking androgen receptors and decreasing androgen production in both the ovaries and adrenal glands.

Strabismus The misalignment of the eye usually referred to as "cross-eye."

Subcutaneous Under the skin.

Superficial/light peel A procedure that removes the top layer of the skin, the epidermis, either with microdermabrasion, glycolic or salycilic acids, or laser. It involves no recovery time and is sometimes called "the lunchtime peel."

Telangiectasia A condition in which red capillaries become increasingly more visible through thinning skin. Affects mostly fair-skinned people. Lasers provide the most effective treatment—they heat the blood vessel, which then coagulates and gets absorbed into the body.

Telomeres Sequences of nucleic acids extending from the ends of chromosomes (like caps). These caps shorten every time a cell divides, which is believed to lead to cellular damage. Each time a cell divides, it duplicates itself a little less perfectly than the time before, eventually leading to cellular dysfunction and aging. Telomerese is the enzyme that can prevent this shortening.

Tendons Cords of fibrous tissue at the end of a muscle that attach the muscle to bone.

Toner An acidic liquid used to wipe the skin after cleansing, to pick up any dirt or makeup traces the cleanser may have missed.

Topical Applied to the skin; not ingested.

Tretinoin An antibiotic that regulates sebaceous release and exfoliates the skin. Some examples are Retin A, Differin, and Accutane.

Triglycerides Tiny particles that comprise body fat and that are predictive of heart disease.

T-zone The area of the forehead, nose, and chin that tends to collect/secrete the most sebaceous oil.

UVA/UVB Ultraviolet rays. Electromagnetic radiation emitted by the sun and some halogen light with wavelengths between 200 nanometers and 400 nanometers. Exposure to excessive UV radiation damages DNA and can cause health problems such as skin cancer.

Veins Blood vessels that carry blood to the heart from other parts of the body.

Water-soluble Dissolves in water.

Zinc oxide A sunscreen that provides the broadest spectrum of protection against harmful UVA/UVB rays.